Active Antimicrobial Food Packaging

Edited by Işıl Var and Sinan Uzunlu

Published in London, United Kingdom

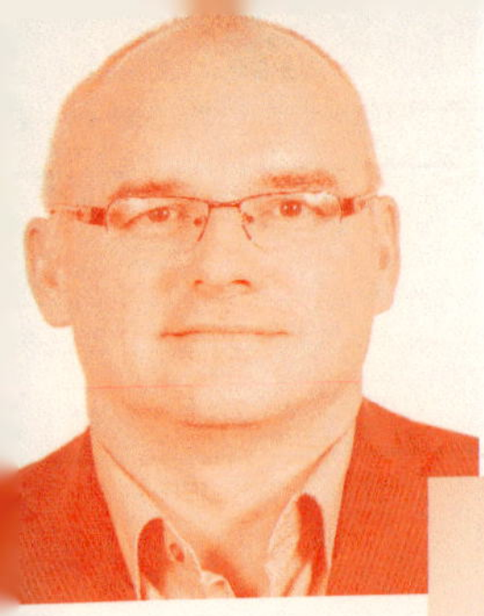
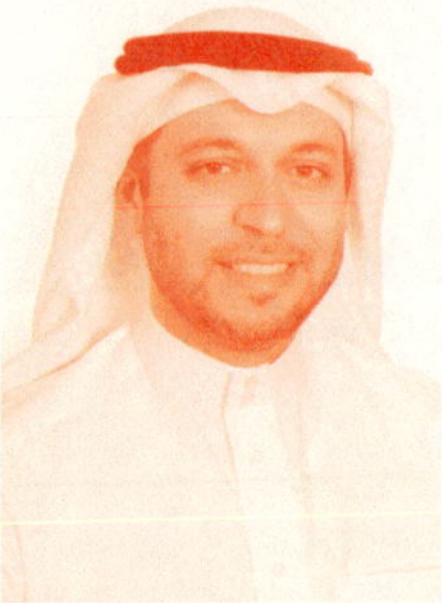
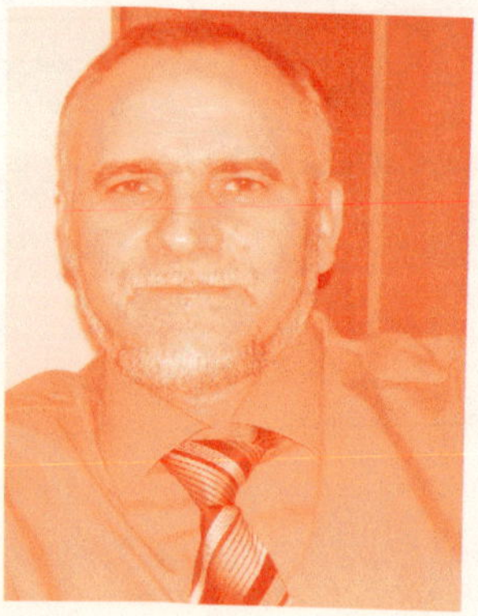
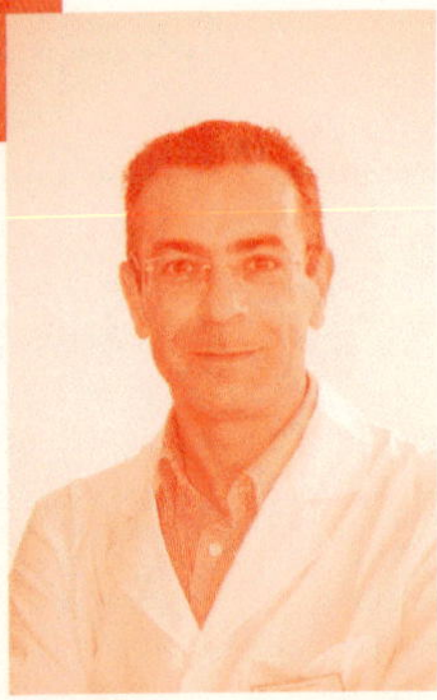
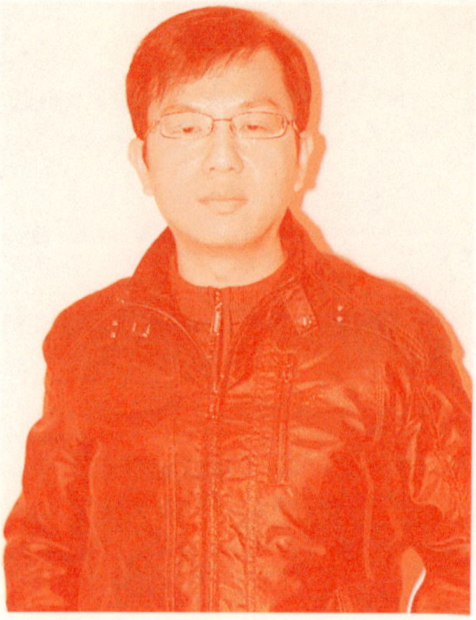
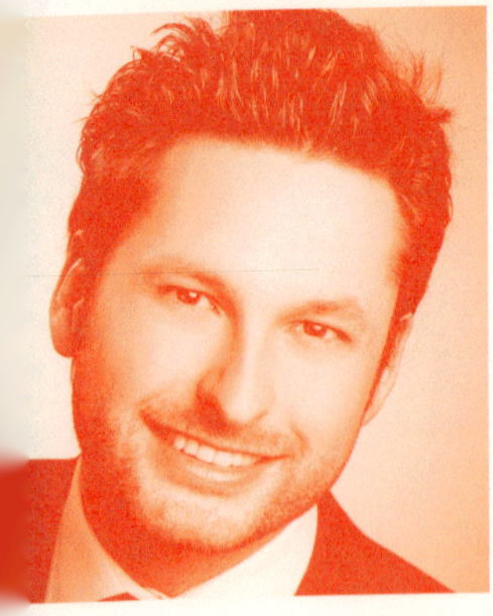
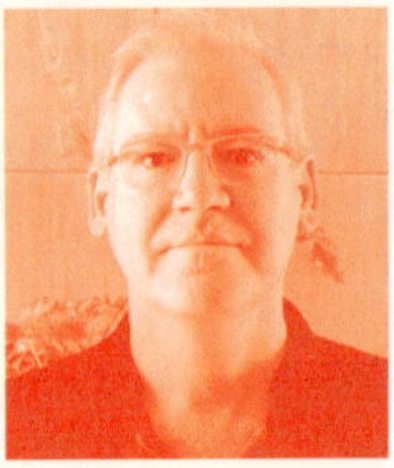

IntechOpen

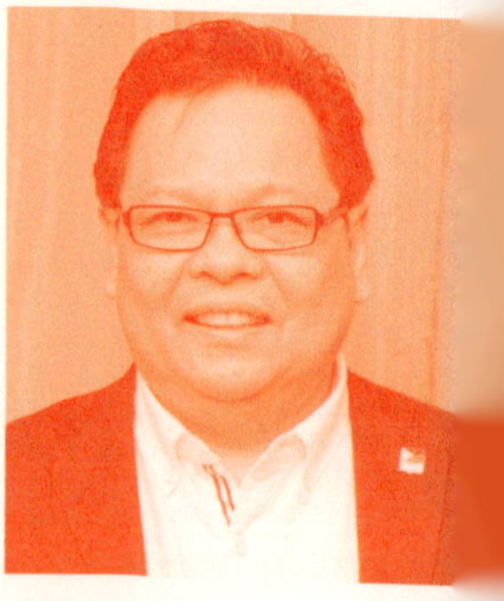
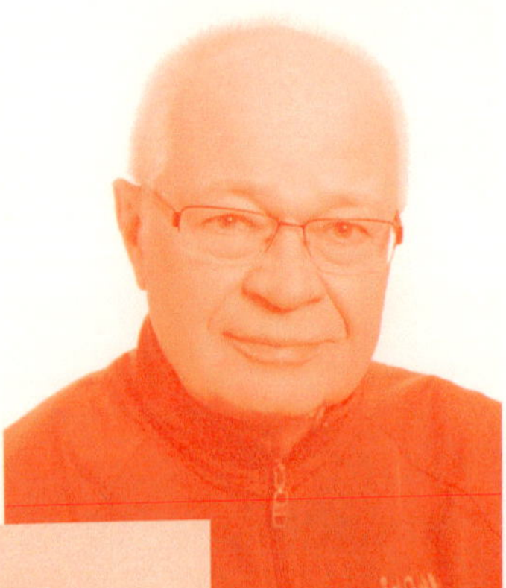
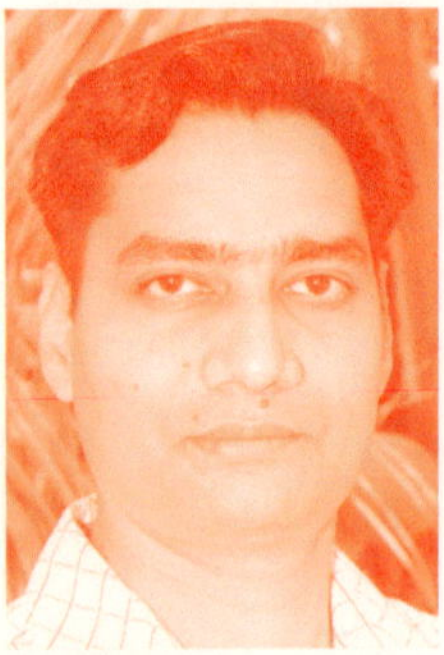
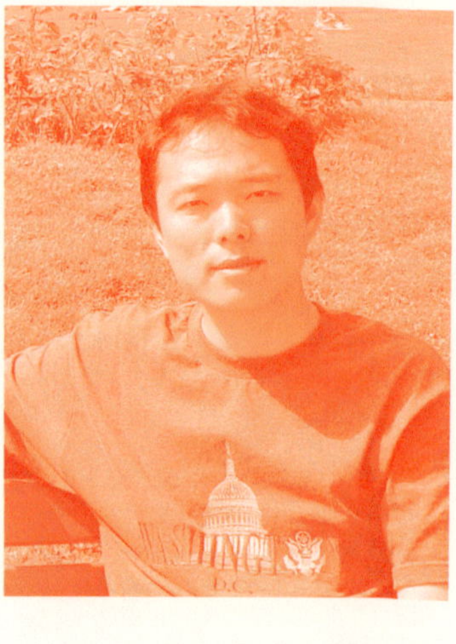
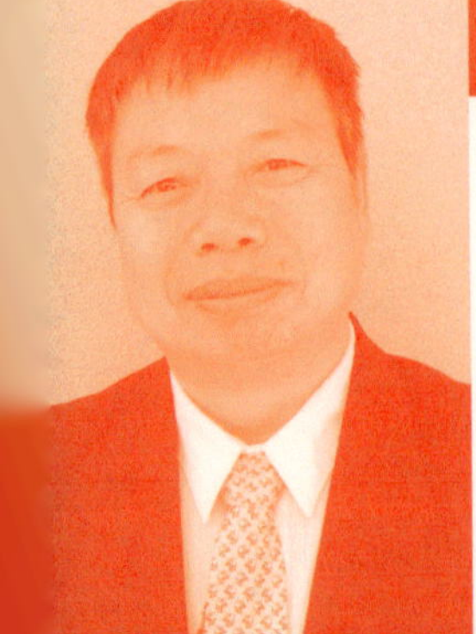
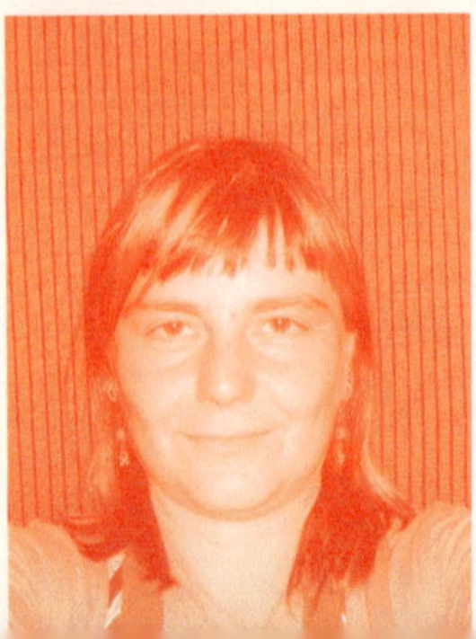

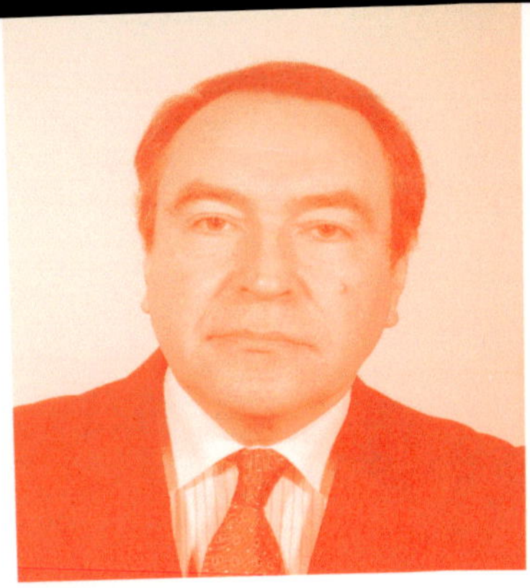

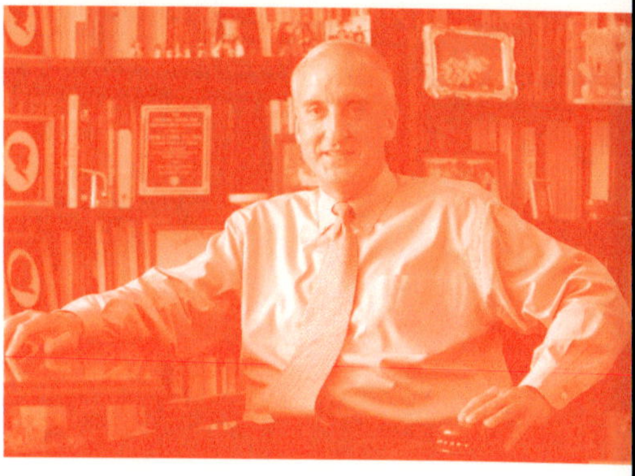

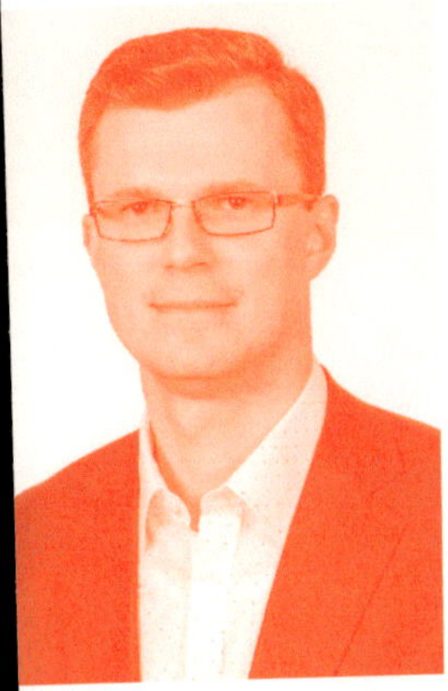

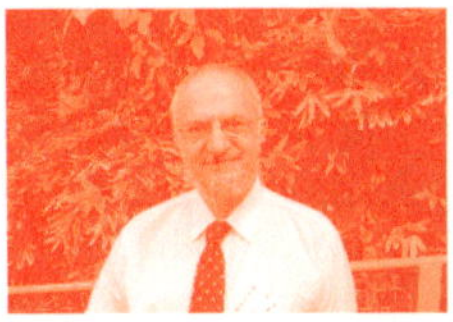

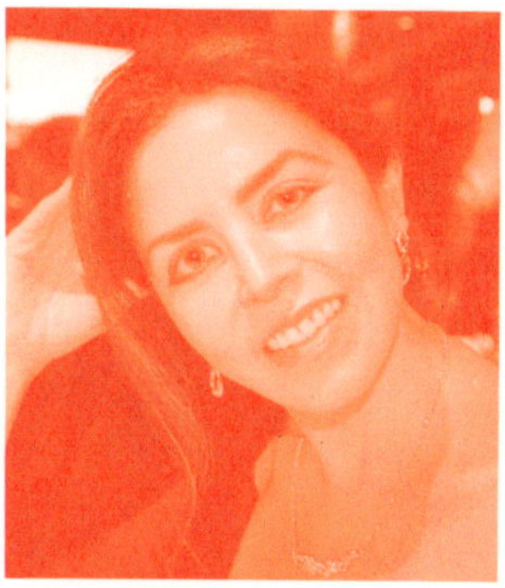

Supporting open minds since 2005

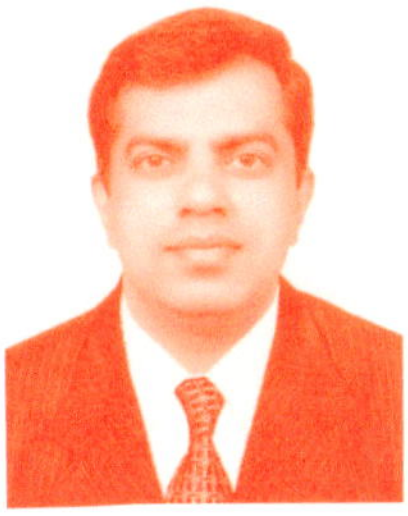

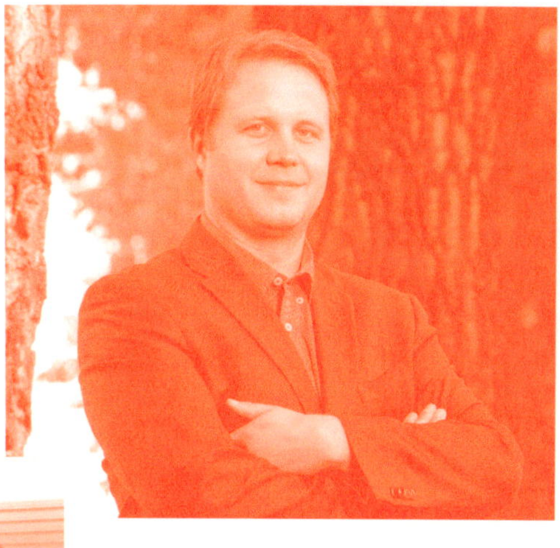

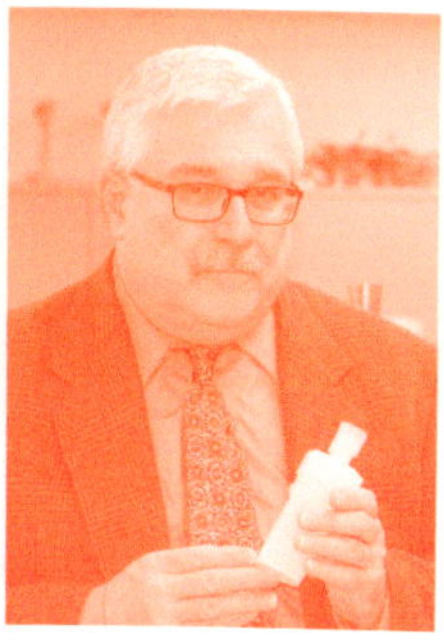

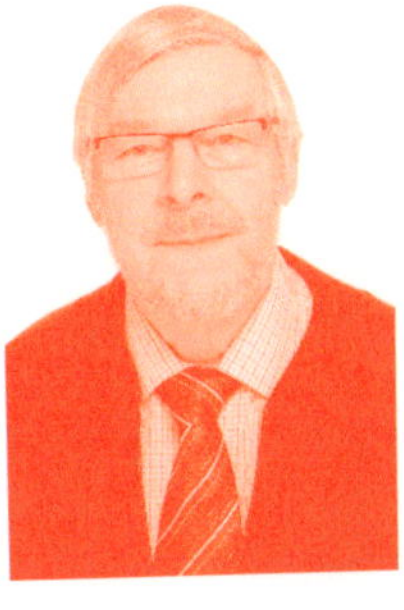

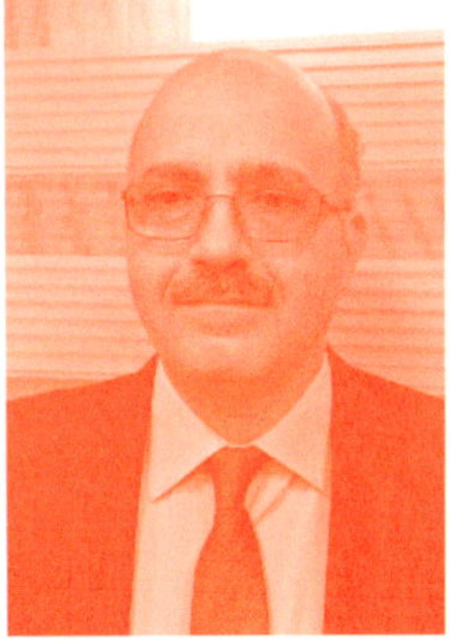

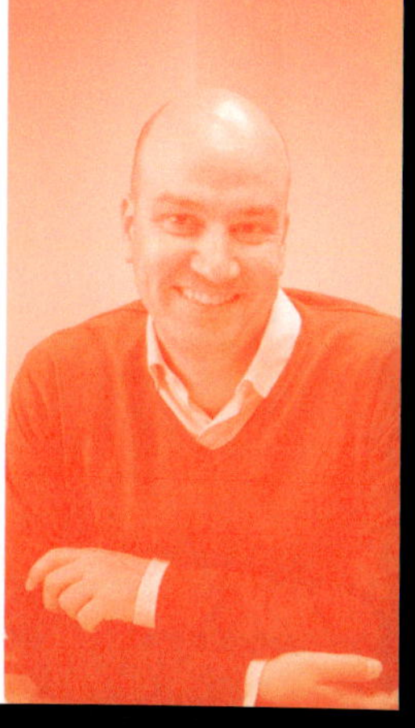

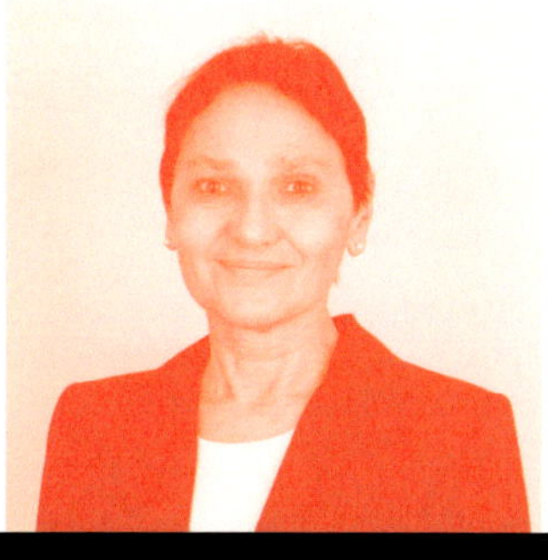

Active Antimicrobial Food Packaging
http://dx.doi.org/10.5772/intechopen.74450
Edited by Işıl Var and Sinan Uzunlu

Contributors
Saroat Rawdkuen, Farhan Saeed, Muhammad Afzaal, Tabussam Tufail, Aftab Ahmed, Norizah Sarbon, Nurul Saadah Saad, Cecilia Rojas, Carlos P. Saenz, Judith A. Rocha, Işıl, Sinan Uzunlu

First published in London, United Kingdom, 2019 by IntechOpen
IntechOpen is the global imprint of INTECHOPEN LIMITED, registered in England and Wales, registration number: 11086078, The Shard, 25th floor, 32 London Bridge Street
London, SE19SG – United Kingdom
Printed in Croatia

British Library Cataloguing-in-Publication Data
A catalogue record for this book is available from the British Library

Additional hard copies can be obtained from orders@intechopen.com

Active Antimicrobial Food Packaging
Edited by Işıl Var and Sinan Uzunlu
p. cm.
Print ISBN 978-1-78985-003-1
Online ISBN 978-1-78985-004-8

For EU product safety concerns:
IN TECH d.o.o., Prolaz Marije Krucifikse Kozulić 3, 51000 Rijeka, Croatia, info@intechopen.com or visit our website at intechopen.com.

Meet the editors

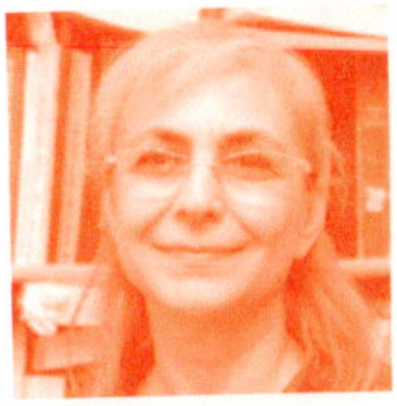

Dr. Işıl Var is a professor in food engineering at Çukurova University, Turkey. She received her BSc in 1981 at Hacettepe University, and MSc in 1987 and PhD in 1993 at Çukurova University. She had a postdoctoral visit to the University of Sussex in the UK between 1993 and 1995. She has published 70 papers in national and international peer-reviewed journals in the field of food microbiology, and filed a patent with Dr. Sinan Uzunlu on modified atmosphere packaging. She has graduated several MSc and PhD students. She is a member of numerous national and international societies. She received several awards from the Scientific and Technological Research Council of Turkey and VTT Technical Research Centre of Finland in 2007.

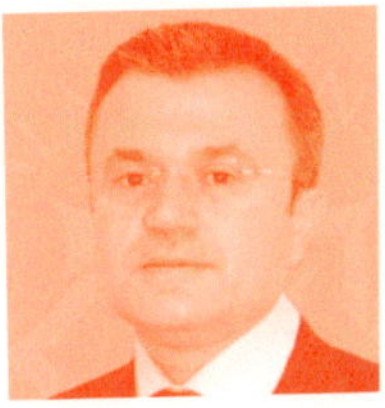

Dr. Sinan Uzunlu is a lecturer in food engineering at Alanya Alaaddin Keykubat University, Turkey. He received his BSc in 1999 at Çukurova University, and MSc in 2002 and PhD in 2012 at Akdeniz and Çukurova universities, respectively. He had postdoctoral visits to the University of Reading in the UK between 2014 and 2017. He has published 13 papers in national and international peer-reviewed journals in the field of food microbiology and food packaging, and filed a patent with Professor Işıl Var on modified atmosphere packaging. He is a member of national and international societies. He has received awards from the Scientific and Technological Research Council of Turkey, the Council of Higher Education (Turkey), and the Society of Chemical Industry (UK).

Contents

Preface

Food packaging is an essential process to obtain a durable good for both producers and consumers. The primary function of packaging is to protect foods from physical, chemical, and biological spoilage during their shelf life. The shelf life period is very much dependent on the conditions of the packaging and storage conditions of the foodstuffs. This period determines not only the stability of the foods but also affects their safety, because marketed foods must be ready to consume in terms of food safety conditions. If the safety of foods isn't sufficient to comply with the quality standards, then public health will be at risk. To overcome such problems the food industry has been implementing many solutions to provide the best marketed foodstuffs. Packaging is one of these attempts. In the current hi-tech world, packaging is experiencing a renewing process to stand up to trends. Therefore, active and intelligent packaging is being researched and marketed by the global packaging community. Active food packaging refers to actively changing the conditions of the packaging within the atmospheric gas composition of the inner and/or outer surface of the package to extend the shelf life of packed foods. Specifically, active antimicrobial packaging uses packaging materials to carry antimicrobials to the food to provide bioactivity in the packaging atmosphere. Intelligent packaging can sense environmental changes and inform the retailer or consumer of the new conditions of the package atmosphere because the conditions might be negatively changed during the transportation or storage periods, for example temperature fluctuation, gas exchange, microbial growth, or off-flavor release. Therefore, this kind of packaging communicates with the end user to display knowledge of ingredients, production, and expiry date.

The current book is composed of five chapters and is aimed at enlightening readers of the adaptation of active food packaging applications. Chapter 1 is an introductory chapter written by the editors of the book, Sinan Uzunlu and Işıl Var. Chapter 2 is written by Farhan Saeed, Muhammad Afzaal, Tabussam Tufail, and Aftab Ahmad. The authors have extensively reviewed the use of natural antimicrobial agents for active packaging applications. Related with that chapter, authors Cecilia Rojas de Gante, Judith A. Rocha, and Carlos P. Saenz Collins have provided their research in Chapter 3. A review by Nurul Saadah Said and Norizah Mhd Sarbon is provided on protein-based active film as antimicrobial food packaging in Chapter 4. The edibility of protective films has been known since the ancient era of human society. Chapter 5 is on edible films incorporated with active compounds, including their properties and application and is authored by Rawdkuen Saroat. We are grateful to all the contributors who made this book possible, and it is our expectation that this book will be beneficial for students, academicians, and professionals in the field of food and materials science, and in the packaging community.

We would like to express our special thanks to Ms. Romina Skomersic, who served as Publishing Process Manager, for her timeless support to finalize the book project.

We also thank the publisher InTechOpen, Pamukkale University, and Çukurova University for their concern and support to publish this book.

Prof. Dr. Işıl Var
Çukurova University Agricultural Faculty Food Engineering Department,
Adana, Turkey

Dr. Sinan Uzunlu
Alanya Alaaddin Keykubat University Rafet Kayış Engineering Faculty Food
Engineering Department,
Alanya-Antalya, Turkey

Chapter 1

Introductory Chapter: Active Antimicrobial Food Packaging

Sinan Uzunlu and Işıl Var

1. Introduction

Food spoilage is the most matter of concern for growers, retailers and consumers; because, foods can be easily deteriorated in a short time unless precautions are taken. Although processing of raw foods by various unit operations preserves the foods up to consumption, the processed foods mostly need to be packaged for a safe retailing and consumption. The basic functions of a food packaging are protection, containment, convenience and communication. However, these are found passive, whereas active functions are needed nowadays [1].

The term 'active packaging' basically refers to shifting protective role of passive packaging to an active role. This means to actively change the conditions of the package within its atmospheric gas composition of inner and/or outer surface of the package to extend the shelf life of packed foods. Antioxidants, enzymes, aromatic compounds, nutraceuticals, essential oils and antimicrobial compounds are used as emitters (active releasing systems) or absorbers (active scavenging systems) in active packaging. European Regulation EC No 450/2009 defines the active packaging as '*deliberately incorporate components that would release or absorb substances into or from the packaged food or the environment surrounding the food*' [1, 2].

Moisture, odour, flavour or gases in the package such as oxygen, carbon dioxide, ethylene are absorbed or emitted by active releasing systems (emitters) or active scavenging systems (absorbers). Active releasing systems are mainly used as antioxidant or antimicrobial carbon dioxide releaser, whereas active scavenging systems (absorbers) are used for oxygen, moisture and ethylene scavenger or absorber [1, 2].

Active releasing systems are using an active compound (green tea extract, tocopherols, butylated hydroxytoluene, citric acid, sodium bicarbonate, etc.), where incorporated to the film or tray structure, while active scavenging systems are using sealed small sachets carrying an active compound (iron, ascorbic acid, photosensitive dyes, palladium, zeolites, etc.) in the packaging. However, the kind of scavenger use in the package is taking concerns for elders and children who might consume the scavengers falsely or the accidental breakage of scavenger sachets might result to an undesired consumption of scavenger material, such as iron, palladium, catechol and oxidative enzymes. It should be outlined that scavenger use in Asian market was positively implemented when compared to European market [2].

Active antimicrobial food packaging is an emerging technology in food packaging, because consumers are demanding more natural foods with less additive usage in the food formulations. In this point, antimicrobial compounds are incorporated into the packaging materials (film and/or tray) or coating onto the packaging surface, or immobilising them in sachets to combat with spoiling microorganisms and pathogens in foods. Therefore, this kind of usage reduces the addition of required amount of active compounds in the food formulations [1].

IntechOpen

Minimal usage versus instant usage of antimicrobials displays equal or higher antimicrobial activity by release mechanism. Another advantage of active packaging is that additives are released in a controlled manner, while using the additives in food formulations might not be fully effective; because, additives could be consumed by reactions in foods. Besides, aerobic microbial spoilers have chance to be effectively controlled, because the volatile antimicrobials are released into the package headspace in vapour phase. Hence, some of the antimicrobials (bacteriocins, enzymes, organic acids, nano-sized metal oxides and bacteriophages) are handled as non-volatile basis agents in active antimicrobial food packaging and need to be directly contacted with the food, whereas volatile agents do not need a direct contact between food and packaging materials. The fact is that antimicrobial activity penetrates every corner of the package and provides surface protection owing to the gaseous characteristic of the agent [3–5].

Essential oils, extracted compounds of various plants or animals, bacteriocins, enzymes, organic acids, nano-sized metal oxides and bacteriophages are commonly studied for use in antimicrobial packaging in numerous researches [3, 4]. Flowers, buds, leaves, stem, bark and seeds are the common materials used for their essential oils (EOs). Plants synthesise two kinds of oils, which are fixed oils and essential oils. Esters of glycerol and fatty acids are defined as fixed oils, whereas EOs are composed of volatile, organic compounds originating from a single botanic source, that provide the flavour and fragrance of the plant [6]. The performance of EOs for antimicrobial and antioxidant activities depends on the plant's botanical characteristics, season, harvesting and extraction conditions, as well as complexity of the foods such as pH, water activity and lipid content affects the performance of EOs, while reproducibility, organoleptic acceptance, migration and allergic reactions of the EOs are limiting factors for use in real packaging conditions [4].

Allergic contact dermatitis is the most common type of adverse reaction of EOs, where cinnamon bark, laurel leaf and tea tree are the reported EOs. The possible toxicity of the EOs is the major concern in food packaging that governed by regulations. Some EOs contain potential eye and airway irritation compounds; therefore, the safety of EOs should be checked when used in food packaging, because EOs are used for their antimicrobial effect in the vapour phase that may result in unwanted respiratory diseases. The reason is, volatile organic compounds are also present in some essential oil constituents and is defined by the US Environmental Protection Agency as '*any compound of carbon, excluding carbon monoxide, carbon dioxide, carbonic acid, metallic carbides, or carbonates, and ammonium carbonate, which participates in atmospheric photochemical reactions*'. In fact, EOs are not a significant cause of respiratory disease; however, inhaled fragrant molecules can trigger attacks in people with asthma or multiple chemical sensitivity. To prevent the EOs-based hazards, limiting the doses and concentrations is a simple and effective way in daily intake. However, in case of the packaging applications, migration limits are important when manufacturing plastics for food contact, where published by European Commission [4, 6].

The research-oriented studies of food scientists and packaging engineers have a leading role in the packaging community. Fabricating an active packaging material is provided by various processing methods that affect film structure and property, which determines the release rate and finally the stability of the active compound. The key word is release rate. The interaction between the packaging material (acted as carrier) and the active compound (acted as releaser) determines the release rate, which have a direct effect on the food quality. The commercial processes of active packaging films involve the cast film and blown film processes. The processing of films follows the order: melting a polymer resin, extruding the polymer melt through a die, stretching and cooling the melted polymer into a film. When required, more than two polymers can be blended using a chaotic mixer [5].

The success of the produced controlled release packaging material is laid on a conceptual framework that determined by Yam and co-workers [5]. The framework is mainly structured on process, structure, property and food parameters. The latter is basically structured on food research, while the formers are structured on packaging research basis. The required shelf life depending on the storage conditions, as well as package contact and the subjected food composition is governed by target release rate of the active compound from packaging material. Stability of active compound/s and release rate, properties of packaging material (e.g. gas permeability) are related with the package structure, morphology of blended polymer and localization of active compounds. These are affected by processing methods such as cast film, blown film, smart blending (chaotic advection), lamination/co-extrusion, solution casting/coating. Type and ratio of the polymer/s and the property of active compound are also determinative in the outlined framework [5].

There are a number of published articles on the current chapter in literature. However, it was our aim to reflect a brief introduction on active antimicrobial food packaging rather than to provide an extensive chapter to the reader. Recently documented reviews for active food packaging by Janjarasskul and Suppakul, Yildirim et al., Ahmed et al. and Ribeiro-Santos et al., as well a review highlighting sachet use in antimicrobial food packaging by Otoni et al. are recommended for further reading [2, 4, 7–10].

The fact is that a number of studies are made by casting method or solvent process to prepare active films in laboratories. Therefore, many of them failed to adapt to the real packaging processes. Some of the reported researches are successfully implemented to the industrial applications [10]. Applications subjected to trade will be summarised in the following statements. An organic compound allyl isothiocyanate (AITC) is used in sheets, labels and films in Japanese market using Wasaouro™ trademark. A bacteriocin, natamycin-based, antifungal coating under the brand name SANICO®, is available for use in cheeses and sausages. Carbon dioxide sachets for use as emitters to provide suppressing microorganism growth and preventing package collapse in modified atmosphere packaging (MAP) is also commercially available under the Verifrais™ brand. However, UltraZap XtendaPak contents have both antimicrobial agents and CO_2 emitter for meat, poultry and seafood packaging. *Salmonella* spp., *Campylobacter* spp. and *Escherichia coli* growth in fresh meat are controlled by using silver nanocomposite films under the brand names Biomaster®, Irgaguard®, Surfacine®, Aglon®, d2p®, Ionpure® and Bactiblock®. An antimicrobial paper, Food-touch®, carrying silver-based additive is used during transportation of fresh fish fillets [8].

In future, to gain the sustainability in active food packaging, tailor-made packaging solutions will be needed for specific food products. Besides, the trend today is using bio-degradable agro-polymers and animal-derived polymers in active food packaging to reduce the waste of packaging materials, especially plastics. This is because of the fact that globally we waste millions of tonnes of plastics in the environment, and those plastic debris threatens the whole ecosystem, which we share with plants and animals [11].

For a sustainable ecosystem, starch, proteins (e.g. casein, whey, soy, gluten, corn maize), polylactic acid, polyhydroxyalkanoate, polyhydroxybutyrate, chitosan are used for their biodegradability both in researches and industrial applications in active packaging [10]. Relatively, high cost and mechanical features of the natural biodegradable polymers versus the synthetic polymers are the limiting factors for their usage in food packaging. However, mechanical performances (tensile strength, elongation at break, etc.) and barrier properties (gases, water vapour) could be increased by blending with common synthetic polymers, such as polyethylene (PE), polypropylene (PP) and plasticizers (water, glycerol, glycol, etc.) [11].

The performance of the polymer blends depends on three main parameters, which are miscibility, compatibility and morphology. The preferred method in industries is melt blending, which is found economic and proper to combine two or more dissimilar characteristics of polymers. Currently, the strategy for compatibilization processes to produce high-performance polymer blends is being undertaken. Therefore, the biodegradable polymers are expected to decrease the amount of conventional polymers usage, such as PE and PP, in the packaging production chain [11].

Apart from this introductory chapter, this book is composed of four chapters and aimed to introduce the reader with active antimicrobial food packaging, as well as regarding concerns of the consumers on food additives. An overview of using natural antimicrobial agents is summarized in Chapter 1, which meet the consumer demands on replacing natural antimicrobials instead of synthetic additive usage in the food industry. Examples for using native plants of Mexico for developing active antimicrobial films are provided in Chapter 2, as an article. Active films, carbohydrates, and proteins as well are used for fabrication. Chapter 3 gives detailed information on protein usage in active antimicrobial food packaging. The use of active compounds in edible films is outlined in Chapter 4.

Author details

Sinan Uzunlu[1]* and Işıl Var[2]

1 School of Applied Sciences, Pamukkale University, Çivril, Turkey

2 Faculty of Agriculture, Department of Food Engineering, Çukurova University, Adana, Turkey

*Address all correspondence to: suzunlu@hotmail.com

References

[1] Yam KL, Lee DS. Emerging food packaging technologies: An overview. In: Yam KL, Lee DS, editors. Emerging Food Packaging Technologies: Principles and Practice. Cambridge (UK): Woodhead Publishing; 2012. pp. 1-9

[2] Yildirim S, Röcker B, Pettersen MK, Nilsen-Nygaard J, Ayhan Z, Rutkaite R, et al. Active packaging applications for food. Comprehensive Reviews in Food Science and Food Safety. 2018;**17**: 165-199. DOI: 10.1111/1541-4337.12322

[3] López-Carballo G, Gómez-Estaca CR, Hernández-Muñoz GR. Active antimicrobial food and beverage packaging. In: Yam KL, Lee DS, editors. Emerging Food Packaging Technologies: Principles and Practice. Cambridge (UK): Woodhead Publishing; 2012. pp. 27-51

[4] Otoni CG, Espitia PJP, Avena-Bustillos RJ, McHugh TH. Trends in antimicrobial food packaging systems: Emitting sachets and absorbent pads. Food Research International. 2016;**83**:60-73. DOI: 10.1016/j.foodres.2016.02.018

[5] Yam KL, Zhu X. Controlled release food and beverage packaging. In: Yam KL, Lee DS, editors. Emerging Food Packaging Technologies: Principles and Practice. Cambridge, London (UK): Woodhead Publishing; 2012. pp. 13-26

[6] Tisserand R, Young R. The respiratory system. In: Essential Oil Safety: A Guide for Health Care Professionals. 2nd ed. London (UK): Churchill Livingstone Elsevier; 2014. pp. 100-109

[7] Janjarasskul T, Suppakul P. Active and intelligent packaging: The indication of quality and safety. Critical Reviews in Food Science and Nutrition. 2018;**58**:808-831. DOI: 10.1080/10408398.2016.1225278

[8] Ahmed I, Lin H, Zou L, Brody AL, Li Z, Qazi IM, et al. A comprehensive review on the application of active packaging technologies to muscle foods. Food Control. 2017;**82**:163-178. DOI: 10.1016/j.foodcont.2017.06.009

[9] Ribeiro-Santos R, Andrade M, Sanches-Silva A. Application of encapsulated essential oils as antimicrobial agents in food packaging. Current Opinion in Food Science. 2017;**14**:78-84

[10] Guilbert S, Gontard N. Agro-polymers for edible and biodegradable films: Review of agricultural polymeric materials, physical and mechanical characteristics. In: Innovations in Food Packaging. London (UK): Elsevier; 2005. pp. 263-276

[11] Muthuraj R, Misra M, Mohanty AK. Biodegradable compatibilized polymer blends for packaging applications: A literature review. Journal of Applied Polymer Science. 2018;**135**:1-35. DOI: 10.1002/app.45726

Chapter 2

Use of Natural Antimicrobial Agents: A Safe Preservation Approach

Farhan Saeed, Muhammad Afzaal, Tabussam Tufail and Aftab Ahmad

Abstract

Microorganism contamination at various stages of food chain is one of the major causes for food spoilage that ultimately leads to food waste, increasing food insecurity issues and substantial economic losses. Various synthetic chemical preservatives are being used to control microbial food spoilage and to extend product shelf life. Researchers and consumers are discouraging the use of synthetic preservatives due to their negative health impacts. Naturally occurring antimicrobials have gained attention among researchers and food manufacturer due to their safety and nontoxic status. Natural preservatives are easy to obtain from plants, animals and microbes. These naturally occurring antimicrobial agents can be isolated from indigenous sources using various advanced techniques. Natural preservatives such as nisin, essential oils, and natamycin have effective potential against spoilage and pathogenic microorganisms. The regulations regarding the use of these naturally occurring preservatives are not well defined in some developing countries. This chapter focuses on source and their potential role, antimicrobial mechanism in food preservation, and current knowledge on the subject.

Keywords: natural antimicrobials, food safety, regulations

1. Introduction

The world population is increasing tremendously and food security is a highly-managed issue as approximately one-third of all produced food for human consumption is either lost or wasted [1]. Due to the lack of advanced handling technologies, developing countries have more postharvest losses as compared to developed countries. It is still an alarming situation in many developing countries as maximum amount of the produce is lost during post-harvest [2], while in industrialized countries one third of the food waste occurred at the retail or consumer levels [1]. The detail of the losses of differ category is as follows; root crops (40–50%), fruits, and vegetables (35%), fish and seafood (30%), cereals (20%), meat, oil seed, and dairy products (20%) [2].

There are many reasons for this massive global food loss but microbial spoilage is the leading cause for this loss. This leads to food spoilage and enhance the food insecurity issues worldwide. Microbial contamination not only causes food loss but also has undesirable effects on the organoleptic product quality.

IntechOpen

Among spoilage microorganisms, bacteria, fungi (yeast and mold) are the major concerns. Fungi are the major cause for food spoilage at any stage of the food chain because of their ability to grow in low moisture and stress physiological conditions [3]. Fungi not only cause the food spoilage they have ability to produce secondary metabolites like mycotoxins that cause serious health issues in humans. These mycotoxins are able to withstand various harsh food processing conditions, the impact of microbial contamination at each level of food chain (Farm to Fork) noticeably lead to huge economic losses for not only producer as well as consumer [1]. Three main stages of microbial contamination routes are; the field (water, soil, and air), raw materials (crops, meats, and milk) and food processing and manufacturing levels. Various methods and technologies can be used to control the contamination at each stage [4].

Chemical preservatives (benzoate, propionate, sorbate, nitrate, nitrite, and sulfites) are widely used to control the microbial growth. Several traditional food-preservation techniques (freezing, chilling, reduction of water activity, modified atmosphere packaging, acidification, nutrient restriction, fermentation, and nonthermal physical treatments or the addition of synthetic antimicrobials) have been utilized to control food spoilage microorganisms [5]. In recent era, it has been noticed that synthetic preservative have raised many health concern issues. Consumers are increasingly aware of the relationship of health issues and the food they consume. The awareness of the consumers are being increasing about the synthetic-based antimicrobials in the food formulations. These additives have serious impacts on human health as their long run use causes liver damage, asthma, many allergic reaction, and even cancer. and these concerns increasing the use of natural Antimicrobials [6].

The use of synthetic preservative is being discouraged by food scientists and consumers due to their harmful impacts on human health [7]. Therefore, scientists are inspired to find alternative natural antimicrobial agents for the preservation of foods. There are two major categories of antimicrobials that are naturally occurring; 1. Combination of different compounds that extracted from different plants and animals or microorganisms with special antimicrobial characteristics. Essential oils, bacteriocins, protamine, endolysins, lysozyme, lactoferrin, flavor compounds, phenolic compounds, chitosan, isothiocyanates and bacteriocins have been applied to fresh and processed fruits and vegetables. The use of probiotics to show antagonistic effect in pathogens have been shown in different in VIVO studies [8].

In this regard plants are being considered as most important and rich natural source of antimicrobial substances like saponins, tannins, alkaloids, alkenyl phenols, glycoalkaloids, flavonoids, sesquiterpenes, lactones, terpenoids and phorbol esters [9]. These plant substances act as antimicrobial, antioxidants, flavor and color enhancer. These properties of the plant agents do not only extend the shelf life of the product but also enhance the organoleptic acceptability of the products. These substances play a vital role in preventing the growth of foodborne pathogens and thus reduce the chances of illness [10]. Additionally, most plant-derived extracts are generally recognized as safe (GRAS) and Qualified Presumption of Safety (QPS) status in the USA and EU, respectively [11]. Natural antimicrobials have wide application and can be applied as preservatives in fruits and vegetables to ensure safety, protect the quality and extend shelf life. These agents can be obtained from animal, plant, and microbial sources, where they play a role in the natural defense system of their hosts.

Due to potential adverse effect of certain synthetic fungicides and preservatives on environment and health there is a strong societal manufacturer and regulatory authorities demand for less processed and synthetic preservative-free foods and the use of natural preservative as alternatives. Such alternatives mainly include natural preservatives from plants, animals, and microorganisms themselves and their metabolites. The use of such natural agents will build the consumer confidence regarding the consumption of food products. These alternatives are complementary to hurdle technologies. However, their use of natural agents for food preservation is not regulated in many countries, and ingestion of some of them raises questions about health effects, especially when consumed over period of time. The objective of this chapter is to focus on the availability of natural antimicrobial agents, their sources, action mechanism, food applications and regulations.

2. Sources and types of natural antimicrobial agents

Natural preservatives can be derived from various sources. However, plants, animals and microorganisms are considered as major source of these essential substances. These derived compounds have wide application to fresh and processed

Plant-based products	Target microorganisms	References
Sage Coriander Allspice Mustard Clove Oregano Cinnamon Rosemary Turmeric Ginger	*E. coli*, *Clostridium botulinum*, *Listeria monocytogenes*, *Pseudomonas spp.*, *Clostridium spp.*, *S. aureus*, *Yersinia enterocolitica*, *Bacillus spp.*, *Salmonella*	[49]
Cardamom Seeds of muscadine Celery seed Poppy Seed s of Anise Grape seeds	*E. coli* O157:H7, *Campylobacter Jejuni* *L. monocytogenes*, Typhimurium	[50]
Bell pepper Chives Broccoli as a vegetable Kale	*S. aureus*, *Enterococcus*, *Pseudomonas*, *Bacillus*, *L. monocytogenes*	[51]
Rind Peel of lemon Cassia Peel and extract of pomegranate	*S. aureus*, *Salmonella infantis*, *E. coli*	[52]
Pomegranate Strawberry Pears	*E. coli* O157:H7, *Salmonella*	[53]

Table 1.
Some selected plant products and their natural antimicrobial potential.

fruits and vegetables to prevent spoilage, shelf life extension and to assure safety of the products. Plants, herbs, and spices have been found to be rich sources of aldehydes, ester terpenoids, phenolics, and sulfur-containing compounds. These natural occurring agents commonly found in roots, flowers, leaves, seeds and bulbs and in other parts of the plants. These substances are produced in defensive mechanism and are helpful for inactivation or inhibition of many microorganisms (bacteria, yeast and molds) [12]. Essential oils (EO) that is obtained from different plants have wide application as food additives are considered as good alternatives to synthetics. A large variety of antimicrobial agents can be obtained from spices [13]. Different parts of plants like flowers, bark, herbs, wood leaves, seeds, buds, twigs, fruits, and roots are good sources of volatile oils. Volatile oils can be obtained from plants and spices by various methods [11]. Boiling water or hot steam is the most commonly used method for commercial production of essential oils. However, other extraction techniques, like the use of microwaves or liquid carbon dioxide, could be also used [14] (**Table 1**).

3. Plant extracts as natural antimicrobial agents

Extracts of plants, herbs and spices are GRAS products that are used for centuries in the food products, for longevity and as a means of flavor. Plants and spice extracts have greatest antimicrobial activity. Antimicrobial activity potential of clove, oregano, cinnamon, and thyme essential oils and components, cinnamaldehyde, eugenol, carvacrol, and thymol have been reported in numerous literature. [12]. Essential oils obtained from spices contain active compounds that exhibit the great antimicrobial potential, like 3-phenylprop-2-enal, 5-isopropyl-2-methylphenol, etc. [15]. The above-mentioned compounds show antimicrobial activity against *Aspergillus* spp., *Escherichia coli, Listeria monocytogenes, Shigella sonnei,* and *Shigella flexneri*. *E. coli* and enterohemorrhagic *E. coli* are found more sensitive to garlic extract than what? Garlic extract has good antimicrobial potential against *S. aureus* and *Salmonella typhimurium.* Other essential oils or extracts from, basil, eucalyptus citrus, bay, lemongrass, rosemary, savory, and tea plants have demonstrated antimicrobial activities against selected microorganisms [16]. The composition of essential oils is affected by geographical areas and the time of harvest. Some plants consist of 85% essential oil; while few plants have only traces [17]. The minor components present in essential oils play a vital role as antimicrobial agents through synergistic effects. The essential oil and minor components presently affect the cell membrane of the bacterial cell. The hydrophobic nature of essential oil makes it an effective agent to inactivate the growth of microorganisms. The release of the bacterial cell contents make it unable to grow and reproduce.

Extracts/compounds obtained from plants	Target spoilage and foodborne microorganisms	References
Thyme EO	*L. monocytogenes*	[54]
Grape seed extract	*S. aureus*	[55]
Cranberry extract	*S. aureus*	[56]
Lemongrass EO	*Salmonella enteritidis*	[57]
Garlic extract	*Salmonella* spp.	[58]

Table 2.
Antimicrobial effect of plant-based preservatives against selected spoilage and foodborne microorganisms.

Essential oil cause inactivation of essential enzymes, coagulation of cytoplasm, disturbance of genetic material and ultimately affect cell viability [13] (**Table 2**).

4. Main antimicrobials from plants

4.1 Eugenol

Eugenol is a volatile phenolic compound. Eugenol is the main extracted constituent (70–90%) of cloves and is responsible for clove aroma. Main sources include clove essential oil, buds, and leaves mainly harvested in Eugenol play a prominent role in dental and oral hygiene preparations. Eugenol is used as flavor, irritant, and sensitizer and can produce local anesthesia. Eugenol-producing dental materials are used in clinical dentistry and are effective against *Salmonella Shigella, Clostridium botulinum*, *Listeria monocytogenes*, and *E. coli* [18].

4.2 Thymol

Thymol is one of the most important essential oils found in thyme. The main monoterpene phenol found in thyme essential oil. It has immunomodulators, antioxidant, antibacterial anti-inflammatory, and antifungal properties Thymol is active against *Salmonella* and *Staphylococcus* bacteria. Inhibition effect is due to damage to membrane integrity of the microorganism which further affects pH homeostasis and equilibrium of inorganic ions [19].

4.3 Aldehydes

Fruits and vegetables contain (hexanal, 2-(E)-hexenal, trans-2-hexenal, and hexyl acetate) lipoxygenase pathway plant products for preservation. These are effective against Gram-negative and Gram-positive bacteria. α,β-unsaturated aldehydes have a broad antimicrobial spectrum and show similar activity against Gram-positive and Gram-negative microorganisms [20].

4.4 Carvacrol

Carvacrol, a phenolic compound, is considered one of the main components of certain EOs that employ antimicrobial activity. Its sources include savory, thyme, and oregano. Carvacrol is reported to have disruptive action on the plasma membrane of intracellular ATP content of *E. coli* O157:H7. In different studies, the importance of the hydrophobicity and its antimicrobial effectiveness has been identified [21].

4.5 Vanillin

Vanillin, a phenolic compound present in vanilla pods. It holds tremendous industrial applications in food, pharmaceuticals, beverages, perfumes and as nutraceuticals. Inhibitory activity against several fungi and pathogenic and food spoilage bacteria including species from *Escherichia*, *Klebsiella*, *Salmonella*, *Bacillus*, *Serratia*, *Staphylococcus*, and *Listeria*, these compounds may be used as preservatives in fruits and vegetables, applied as vapors in storage operations or in modified atmosphere packaging [22].

4.6 Allicin

Allicin has biological properties. It is a sulfur-containing natural compound. It has typical smell and taste in freshly cut or crushed garlic. For industrial purpose it is mainly extracted from garlic.

The major physiological role of garlic are its antimicrobial, antioxidant, anticancer, antifibrinolytic, and antiplatelet aggregatory activity has been observed [23].

4.7 Cinnamaldehyde

Cinnamaldehyde is the organic and major active constituent in cinnamon. Cinnamaldehyde has yellowish appearance and is mainly present in the essential oils of cinnamon.

4.8 Alkaloids

Alkaloids are a group of naturally occurring chemical compounds which mostly contain basic nitrogen atoms [24].

4.9 Anti-microbial peptide

Plant antimicrobial peptides act as natural defense compounds against many pathogens (pAMPs) and were discovered in 1942. Potato defensin, hevein, thionines, snakins are the examples of the plant antimicrobial peptides. These act as membrane-active antifungals, antibacterials, and antivirals.

4.10 Citral

Citral is a terpenoid that is oxygenated derivative of terpenes, which is compound of a mixture of two isomers. The trans isomer is known as geranial or citral A. The cis-isomer is known as neral or citral. It has antifungal properties. The antifungal effects of citral and eugenol, has been studied in many research [25].

4.11 Saponins

Saponins are high molecular weight glycosides that are present in a diversity of plants and some marine organisms. They act as an antiviral, as an antimicrobial, as an anticancer drug and when included in animals feeds as a growth stimulatory supplement [25].

4.12 Flavonoids

Flavonoids have been extensively researched are hydroxylated phenolic substances but occur as a C6-C3 unit linked to an aromatic ring. These mainly occur in green teas. The term flavonoid includes the polyphenols, flavanones, flavones, flavan-3-ols, flavonols and anthocyanins. Flavonoids are secondary metabolites well documented for their biological effects, in vitro to be effective antimicrobial substances against a wide array of microorganisms. Flavonoids have good antimutagenic, anti-inflammatory, anticancer, and antiviral, activities. The antimicrobial activity of polyphenols found in fruit, vegetables, and medicinal plants has been extensively investigated against a wide range of microorganisms [26].

4.13 Quinones

Quinones are aromatic rings with two ketone substitutions. They are highly reactive and ubiquitous in nature. Quinones may also render substrates unavailable to the microorganism. Tertiary butylhydroquinone (TBHQ) are approved as food antioxidants to prevent rancidity in fats, oils, and lipid foods.

4.14 Tannins

Polymeric phenolic substances capable of tanning leather or precipitating gelatin from solution, a property known as astringency. Ellagitannin with molecular weights ranging from 500 to 3000 is an excellent example of tannin. Ellagitannin is a general descriptive name for a group of tannin. Ellagitannins are almost found in different parts of the plants including bark, wood, leaves, fruits, and roots. Condensed tannins have shown antimicrobial activities against *E. coli, S. aureus, Salmonella typhimurium, B. subtilis, Shigella sonnei, MDR E. coli, C. albicans,* and *K. pneumonia*. They act by binding the cell wall of bacteria and inhibit their growth.

4.15 Coumarins

Coumarins are phenolic substances made of fused benzene and an alpha pyrone ring. Their antimicrobial activity is directed against fungi, but they also have an effect on bacteria.

4.16 Caffeic acid

Caffeic acid (3,4-dihydroxycinnamic acid) is a simple phenolic acid derived from the hydroxycinnamic acid, with some interesting biological properties, such as antibacterial, fungicide, and antioxidant. The antibacterial activity against *S. epidermidis, S. aureus, and K. pneumoniae*, has been observed 3.3.**Main.**

5. Main antimicrobials from animal origin

5.1 Chitosan

Chitosan is obtained from partial deacetylation of chitin and sometimes known as deacetylated chitin. It is a natural polycationic linear polysaccharide mainly found in shells of marine crustaceans [27]. Due to its nontoxicity biodegradability and low allergenicity have wide application. It has antitumor, antifungal, antimicrobial antioxidant activities [28]. It is effective against Gram-negative bacteria like *Bacteroides fragilis, cholera, Shigella dysenteriae, E. coli, and Vibrio.* Chitosan has good antimicrobial resistance to swelling and antioxidant potential.

5.2 Defensin

These are small cationic peptides and are primarily known for their antimicrobial activities mainly antibacterial and antimycotic. These are found in all mammal s cells and tissues abundant in leukocytes [29].

5.3 Lactoperoxidase

Lactoperoxidase (LP) belongs to peroxidase family, and its primary function is to catalyze the oxidation of certain molecules. It is a group of natural enzymes, widely distributed in nature and found in plants and animals, including man. Lactoperoxidase (LP) secreted by ductal epithelial cells of the mammary gland. The level of LP in bovine milk is about 20 times higher than that of human milk and changes constantly during the postpartum period. Thiocyanate, which is present in significant amounts in saliva, milk, and airway secretion system, is required for the antimicrobial activity. Bacteria *including salmonellae, Shigella, pseudomonads, and coliforms* are not only inhibited by lactoperoxidase (LP) but may be killed [30].

5.4 Lysozyme

It is a single chain polypeptide of 129 amino acids naturally present in bodily secretions such as tears, saliva, and milk. It has good antimicrobial effectiveness and cause death of bacteria by cleaving a glycosidic linkage of bacterial cell walls peptidoglycan. Lysozyme is an important defense mechanism and is considered a part of the innate immune system in most mammals [31], and is also an important component of human breast milk [32]. Large amounts of lysozyme can be found in egg white [33].

5.5 Lactoferrin

Lactoferrin (LF) is iron-binding and bioactive glycoprotein also termed as lactosiderophilin or lactotransferrin. Lactoferrin is present in many body secretions (reproductive, digestive, and respiratory) such as those from the systems. It is present in large amount in bovine colostrum than in mature milk, lactoferrin shows strong antimicrobial effects against various Gram-negative and -positive bacteria, fungi, and parasites. It has been shown to have direct effects on different pathogenic microorganisms including bacteriostatic. [34].

5.6 Avidin

Avidin is a positively charged glycoprotein which is present in egg. Egg also contains biotin. Avidin binds biotin (avidin-biotin system as a diagnostic tool in immunoassays) and makes it unavailable for the use of microorganism. The activity of *E. coli, Klebsiella pneumoniae, Serratia marcescens,* and *P. aeruginosa can be controlled* [35].

5.7 Pleurocidin

It is an antimicrobial peptide consisting of 25 amino acids and is very active against bacteria both Gram-positive and Gram-negative. It has potential for use in food applications due to heat-stability, salt tolerant ability and other characteristics. In many studies it has been found to be effective against many pathogenic organisms like *E. coli* O157:H7, *Vibrio parahaemolyticus, and L. monocytogenes.* [36].

5.8 Protamine

Protamine is a cationic antimicrobial peptide (CAP), used as a natural food preservative. It is obtained from various kinds of fish. It has wide potential for food application due to high stability under heat and a preservative effect in neutral or alkaline food. Protamine does not influence the sensorial characteristics (texture, smell, or taste) of the food to which it is added [37]. It is effective against any gram positive and negative bacteria also useful against yeast and mold as well [38].

5.9 Lactolipids

Lipids may serve to inhibit multiplication and proliferation of disease causing microorganism. The effects increased when used in combination with other antimicrobial agents like lactoglobulins, lactoferrin and lactoperoxidase [39]. Lipids derived from animal origin have good antimicrobial potential against wide range of pathogenic microorganisms. Free fatty acids have been shown to be effective against *S. aureus* and many Gram-positive bacteria like *S. aureus, C. botulinum*, and *L. monocytogenes*. The majority of the lipids derived from animal origin are considered as GRAS and effective for food applications. A projected application of these animal based antimicrobial lipids has been made in infant formulas. This provides protection after hydrolysis of the triglycerides in the gastrointestinal tract (GIT) following consumption [40].

6. Main antimicrobials from microbial origin

6.1 Natamycin

Natamycin has been used food preservation against the food spoilage organisms particularly yeast or mold. Its molecular weight is 665.7 Da. Natamycin is produced by *Streptomyces natalensis* and is effective against almost all molds and yeasts. It has been observed that, however, natamycin has little or no activity against many pathogenic bacteria. Due to its antifungal nature, it has been used in various products like dairy, meats, and many others. Natamycin is effective for juices in both cases (unpasteurized and pasteurized) against growth of yeasts and molds (**Table 3**).

6.2 Reuterin

It is an antimicrobial compound produced by *Lacotobacillus reuteri*. It is water soluble non proteinaceous with a broad antimicrobial range. It is effective against Gram-negative and Gram-positive bacteria filamentous (mold) and nonfilamentous (yeasts). It is active to wide range of pH and resistant to various enzymes like proteolytic and lipolytic. [41]. It exhibit bacteriostatic activity against many pathogenic bacteria particularly against *Listeria monocytogenes*.

6.3 Bacteriophages

Natural bio preservatives from animal and plant origin are considered as alternative to chemical preservatives because of the good hygienic quality, safety and extension of shelf life of food products [42]. Compounds of plants, animals, and microorganism origins are used as natural preservatives because of their cost-effective approach. Both bacteriophages and bacteria can be used as preservatives for food applications. These can be easily propagated. It has been observed that bacteriophage (phages) is favorable because phage has the ability to target specific bacteria [43] (**Table 4**).

Natamycin dosage levels	Method of application	Foods	References
1250–2000 ppm	• Surface treatment • Direct addition • Immersion • coating emulsion	Cheese	[59]
1250–2000 ppm	• Immersion method • Surface treatment by spray	Meat products	
5–10 ppm	• By surface treatment By direct addition	Yogurt	
1250–2000 ppm	• Surface treatment by spray	Bakery products	
7.5 ppm	• Direct addition	Tomato purée/ paste	
2.5–10 ppm	• Direct addition	Fruit juice	

Table 3.
Application of natamycin in different foods as natural antimicrobial agents.

Effective concentration (mg/l) of chitosan	Selected microorganisms	References
2500	*P. aeruginosa*	[60]
150	*Listeria monocytogenes*	
50	*Staphylococcus aureus*	
1500	*Salmonella typhimurium*	
600	*E. coli*	[61]
600	*S. typhi*	
100	*Escherichia coli*	

Table 4.
Antimicrobial potential chitosan (animal-based antimicrobial) agent against different foodborne microorganisms.

6.4 Lactic acid bacteria (LAB)

Lactic acid bacteria are important probiotics that confer many health benefits including protective role in foods. They act as preservative and inhibit the growth of many pathogenic bacteria. They inhibit the growth of pathogen by producing antimicrobial agents like organic acids and bacteriocins (antimicrobial peptides) [44]. Various strains of the bacteria are effective against many pathogens (**Table 5**).

6.5 Bacteriocins

Main antimicrobial compounds produced by many gram positive bacteria. These are actually metabolites of the LAB that are produced during their growth. These polypeptides give the producing microorganism a competitive advantage over other type of microorganisms. Bacteriocins are classified based on their chemical nature and mainly produced by Gram-positive bacteria [45] (**Table 6**).

LAB strain	Target spoilage and foodborne microorganisms	References
Lactobacillus sakei	*Spoilage microorganisms*	[62]
Lactobacillus curvatus	*Spoilage microorganisms*	[63]
L.. curvatus	*Food borne pathogens: Escherichia coli* O157:H7	[64]
Carnobacterium divergens	*L. monocytogenes*	[65]
Enterococcus faecium, Lactococcus lactis	*Listeria innocua and spoilage*	[66]

Table 5.
Antimicrobial effect of LAB against selected spoilage and foodborne microorganisms.

Classification	Target microorganism	References
Lactacin B enterococci	*L. acidophilus Lactobacilli, Lactococcus lactis*	[67]
Lacticin F	*L. acidophilus, Lactobacilli*	[68]
Nisin	*L. lactis subsp lactis*	[69]
Lacticin 3147	*L. lactis subsp lactis*	

Table 6.
Lactic acid bacteria (LAB) as a source of bacteriocins.

6.6 Methods for the extraction of natural antimicrobial agents

The extraction of plant-based antimicrobial with the use of solvents (hydrochloric acid, ammonium chloride, ethanol, methanol, and alcohol) is time consuming and unwieldly. These methods required large amount of solvents and not cost effective regarding economic aspects. In addition the heat treatments can change the activity of bioactive agents [46]. These methods can also change the common natural characteristics, functionality, total content and activity of the compounds. The proposed methods are: direct, aqueous, and juice extraction—have been used widely to study the antimicrobial activity of plant extracts [47].

6.7 Mechanisms of action of natural antimicrobial agents

The action mechanism of natural preservative has not been fully understood. Different natural antimicrobial agents act in different way. In order to understand their mechanism below is the list of possible actions of the natural antimicrobial agents. They target the pathogenic microorganism in one or more of the following ways: membrane-disrupting compounds, direct pH reduction of the substrate, organic acids inhibiting NADH oxidation, organic acids interfering with membrane, and essential oils (EOs) producing structural and functional damage to the bacterial cell membrane.

6.8 Methods for application

Many factors can influence the application of natural antimicrobial agents to food including designing of food, physicochemical properties of food and agents, food composition, different processing operations storage conditions, target microorganism. The application can also influence the sensory, quality and safety aspects of the subjected foods. Sometime natural antimicrobials agents from different sources can transfer odors and flavors to the food. It has been noted that different food constituents like proteins, lipids, complex carbohydrates, and sugars reduce antimicrobial activity. Many methods are available for the application of naturally occurring agents like Edible films, encapsulation and direct methods (spraying, dusting, and dipping).

6.9 Consumer concerns

Natural antimicrobial agents derived from plants, animals and microbial origins are considered safe as compared to synthetic preservatives. The growth of foodborne pathogens has not been observed with the use of natural preservatives. However, the optimal range of plant, animal and microbial based antimicrobials agents need to be defined to avoid any quality and safety issue. Many factors need to be addressed like temperatures, agents, food characteristics, and composition [48]. Preservation by lactic acid bacteria is being considered as natural solution for the preservation of the food commodities. Consumer, manufacturer and researcher giving it more consideration as these natural antimicrobial agents will be good way forward to extend the shelf life and in presentation of food spoilage. Several products composed of bacteria, fungi, and yeasts are currently commercialized worldwide.

7. Conclusion

With the increasing demand of fresh, semi processed, processed and raw food commodities their safety quality and preservation issues are need to be addressed. The regulation and new method of application of natural antimicrobials agents are important factors that should be addressed. Optimization of application methods and regulation will enhance the consumer confidence. The application methods for the natural antimicrobial agents to different food products required higher efficiency. The use of natural antimicrobials on fruits and vegetables without destructively affecting the sensorial characteristics is still a challenge for researchers. To inhibit the growth of spoilage or eliminate pathogenic bacteria, the required concentrations of natural antimicrobial agents is very high. These high concentrations can not only affects sensory qualities but can also have negative impact on human health. Research need to be done on the synergistic combinations of natural antimicrobial agents. A combination of different treatments strongly ensures the safety and quality issues of the food products.

Author details

Farhan Saeed, Muhammad Afzaal*, Tabussam Tufail and Aftab Ahmad
Institute of Home & Food Sciences, Government College University, Faisalabad, Pakistan

*Address all correspondence to: muhammadafzaal@gcuf.edu.pk

References

[1] Gustavsson J, Cederberg C, Sonesson U. Global Food Losses and Food Waste: Extent, Causes and Prevention. Rome, Italy: Food and Agriculture Organization of the United Nations; 2011. p. 9; ISBN 978-92-5-107205

[2] FAO. Save food: Global initiative on food loss and waste reduction—Key findings. Available online: http://www.fao.org/save-food/resources/keyfindings/en/ [Accessed: 2 May 2017]

[3] Kitinoja L, Saran S, Roy SK, Kader AA. Postharvest technology for developing countries: Challenges and opportunities in research, outreach and advocacy. Journal of the Science of Food and Agriculture. 2011;**91**:597-603

[4] Dijksterhuis J, Houbraken J, Samson RA. 2 fungal spoilage of crops and food. In: Kempken F, editor. Agricultural Applications. Berlin/Heidelberg, Germany: Springer; 2013. pp. 35-56, ISBN 978-3-642-36821-9

[5] Davidson PM, Naidu AS. Phyto-phenols. In: Naidu AS, editor. Natural Food Antimicrobial Systems. Boca Raton, FL: CRC Press; 2000. pp. 265-294

[6] Rico D, Martin-Diana AB, Barat JM, Barry-Ryan C. Extending and measuring the quality of fresh-cut fruit and vegetables: A review. Trends in Food Science & Technology. 2007;**18**(7):373-386

[7] Sofos JN, Geornaras I. Overview of current meat hygiene and safety risks and summary of recent studies on biofilms, and control of *Escherichia coli* O157: H7 in nonintact, and *Listeria monocytogenes* in ready-to-eat, meat products. Meat Science. 2010;**86**(1):2-14

[8] Gálvez A, Abriouel H, Benomar N, Lucas R. Microbial antagonists to food-borne pathogens and biocontrol. Current Opinion in Biotechnology. 2010;**21**(2):142-148

[9] Tajkarimi MM, Ibrahim SA, Cliver DO. Antimicrobial herb and spice compounds in food. Food Control. 2010; **21**(9):1199-1218

[10] Rohani SMR, Moradi M, Mehdizadeh T, Saei-Dehkordi SS, Griffiths MW. The effect of nisin and garlic (*Allium sativum* L.) essential oil separately and in combination on the growth of *Listeria monocytogenes*. LWT-Food Science and Technology. 2011; **44**(10):2260-2265

[11] Burt S. Essential oils: Their antibacterial properties and potential applications in foods—A review. International Journal of Food Microbiology. 2004;**94**(3):223-253

[12] Davidson PM, Critzer FJ, Matthew Taylor T. Naturally occurring antimicrobials for minimally processed foods. Annual Review of Food Science and Technology. 2013;**4**:163-190

[13] González-Aguilar GA, Valenzuela-Soto E, Lizardi-Mendoza J, Goycoolea F, Martínez-Téllez MA, Villegas-Ochoa MA, et al. Effect of chitosan coating in preventing deterioration and preserving the quality of fresh-cut papaya 'Maradol'. Journal of the Science of Food and Agriculture. 2009;**89**(1):15-23

[14] Bakkali F, Averbeck S, Averbeck D, Idaomar M. Biological effects of essential oils—A review. Food and Chemical Toxicology. 2008;**46**(2):446-475

[15] Weerakkody NS, Caffin N, Turner MS, Dykes GA. In vitro antimicrobial activity of less-utilized spice and herb extracts against selected food-borne bacteria. Food Control. 2010;**21**(10):1408-1414

[16] Moreira MR, Ponce AG, Del Valle CE, Roura SI. Inhibitory parameters of essential oils to reduce a foodborne pathogen. LWT-Food Science and Technology. 2005;**38**(5):565-570

[17] Bauer K, Garbe D, Surburg H. Natural raw materials in the flavor and fragrance industry. In: Common Fragrance and Flavor Materials: Preparation, Properties and Uses. 4th ed. 2001. pp. 167-226

[18] Ceylan E, Fung DYC. Antimicrobial activity of spices. Journal of Rapid Methods & Automation in Microbiology. 2004;**12**(1):1-55

[19] Lambert RJW, Skandamis PN, Coote PJ, Nychas G-JE. A study of the minimum inhibitory concentration and mode of action of oregano essential oil, thymol and carvacrol. Journal of Applied Microbiology. 2001;**91**(3): 453-462

[20] Bisignano G, Laganà MG, Trombetta D, Arena S, Nostro A, Uccella N, et al. In vitro antibacterial activity of some aliphatic aldehydes from *Olea europaea* L. FEMS Microbiology Letters. 2001;**198**(1):9-13

[21] Ben Arfa A, Combes S, Preziosi-Belloy L, Gontard N, Chalier P. Antimicrobial activity of carvacrol related to its chemical structure. Letters in Applied Microbiology. 2006;**43**(2): 149-154

[22] Fitzgerald DJ, Stratford M, Gasson MJ, Ueckert J, Bos A, Narbad A. Mode of antimicrobial action of vanillin against *Escherichia coli*, *Lactobacillus plantarum* and *Listeria innocua*. Journal of Applied Microbiology. 2004;**97**(1):104-113

[23] Santhosha SG, Jamuna P, Prabhavathi SN. Bioactive components of garlic and their physiological role in health maintenance: A review. Food Bioscience. 2013;**3**:59-74

[24] Ooi LSM, Li Y, Kam S-L, Wang H, Wong EYL, Ooi VEC. Antimicrobial activities of cinnamon oil and cinnamaldehyde from the Chinese medicinal herb *Cinnamomum cassia* Blume. The American Journal of Chinese Medicine. 2006;**34**(03):511-522

[25] Lenardao EJ, Ferreira PC, Jacob RG, Perin G, Leite FPL. Solvent-free conjugated addition of thiols to citral using KF/alumina: Preparation of 3-thioorganylcitronellals, potential antimicrobial agents. Tetrahedron Letters. 2007;**48**(38):6763-6766

[26] Manach C, Scalbert A, Morand C, Rémésy C, Jiménez L. Polyphenols: Food sources and bioavailability. The American Journal of Clinical Nutrition. 2004;**79**(5):727-747

[27] Chandy T, Sharma CP. Chitosan-as a biomaterial. Biomaterials, Artificial Cells, and Artificial Organs. 1990;**18**: 1-24. DOI: 10.3109/10731199009117286

[28] Ngo DH, Kim SK. Chapter Two— Antioxidant effects of chitin, chitosan, and their derivatives. In: Kim SK, editor. Advances in Food and Nutrition Research. Vol. 73. Waltham, MA, USA: Academic Press; 2014. p. 15

[29] Agerberth B, Charo J, Werr J, Olsson B, Idali F, Lindbom L, et al. The human antimicrobial and chemotactic peptides LL-37 and alphadefensins are expressed by specific lymphocyte and monocyte populations. Blood. 2000;**96**: 3086-3093

[30] Reiter B, HaÈrnulv G. Lactoperoxidase antibacterial system: Natural occurrence, biological functions and practical applications. Journal of Food Protection. 1984;**47**:724-732

[31] Varahan S, Iyer VS, Moore WT, Hancock LE. Eep confers lysozyme resistance to enterococcus faecalis via the activation of the extracytoplasmic

function sigma factor sig V. Journal of Bacteriology. 2013;**195**:3125-3134

[32] Lonnerdal B. Nutritional and physiologic significance of human milk proteins. The American Journal of Clinical Nutrition. 2003;**77**:1537S-11543S

[33] Williams S, Vocadlo D. Glycoside hydrolase family 22. Cazypedia. Retrieved 11 April 2017

[34] Al-Nabulsi AA, Holley RA. Effect of bovinelactoferrin against *Carnobacterium viridans*. Bioresource Technology. 2005;**22**:179-187

[35] Korpela J. Avidin, a high affinity biotin-binding protein as a tool and subject of biological research. Medical Biology. 1984;**62**:5-26

[36] Cole A, Darouiche R, Legarda D, Connell N, Diamond G. Characterization of a fish antimicrobial peptide: Gene expression, subcellular localization and spectrum of activity. Antimicrobial Agents and Chemotherapy. 2000;**44**:2039-2045

[37] Burrowes OJ, Hadjicharalambous C, Diamond G, Lee TC. Evaluation of antimicrobial spectrumand cytotoxic activity of pleurocidin for food applications. Journal of Food Science. 2004;**69**(3):66-71

[38] Burton E, Gawande PV, Yakandawala N, LoVetri K, Zhanel GG, Romeo T, et al. Antibiofilm activity of Glm U enzyme inhibitors against catheter-associated uropathogens. Antimicrobial Agents and Chemotherapy. 2006;**50**(5):1835-1840

[39] Mandel ID, Ellison SA. The biological significance of the non immunoglobulin defense factors. In: Pruitt KM, Tenovuo JO, editors. The Lactoperoxidase System Chemistry and Biological Significance. New York: Marcel Dekker; 1985. pp. 1-14

[40] Isaacs CE, Litov RE, Thormar H. Antimicrobial activity of lipids added to human milk, infant formula, and bovine milk. The Journal of Nutritional Biochemistry. 1995;**6**:362-366

[41] El-Ziney MG, van den Tempel T, Debevere JM, Jakobsen M. Application of reuterin produced by *Lactobacillus reuteri* 12002 for meat decontamination and preservation. Journal of Food Protection. 1294; **1999**(62):257-261

[42] Juneja VK, Dwivedi HP, Yan X. Novel natural food antimicrobials. Annual Review of Food Science and Technology. 2012;**3**:381-403

[43] Anany H, Brovko LY, El-Arabi T, Griffiths MW. Bacteriophages as antimicrobials in food products: History, biology and application. In: Handbook of Natural Antimicrobials for Food Safety and Quality. US: Woodhead Publishing; 2014. p. 69

[44] Rydlo T, Miltz J, Mor A. Eukaryotic antimicrobial peptides: Promises and premises in food safety. Journal of Food Science. 2006;**71**(9)

[45] Ricke SC. Anaerobic microbiology laboratory training and writing comprehension for food safety education. In: Food Safety. 2015. pp. 395-419

[46] Herrero M, Cifuentes A, Ibañez E. Sub-and supercritical fluid extraction of functional ingredients from different natural sources: Plants, food-by-products, algae and microalgae: A review. Food Chemistry. 2006;**98**(1): 136-148

[47] Mau J-L, Chen C-P, Hsieh P-C. Antimicrobial effect of extracts from

Chinese chive, cinnamon, and corni fructus. Journal of Agricultural and Food Chemistry. 2001;**49**(1):183-188

[48] An JH. Antimicrobial food packaging. In: Novel Food Packaging Techniques. Vol. 8. 2003. pp. 50-70

[49] Ceylan E, Fung DYC, Sabah JR. Antimicrobial activity and synergistic effect of cinnamon with sodium benzoate or potassium sorbate in controlling *Escherichia coli* O157:H7 in apple juice. Journal of Food Science. 2004;**69**(4):FMS102-FMS106

[50] Ayaz FA, Hayirlioglu-Ayaz S, Alpay-Karaoglu S, Gruz J, Valentova K, Ulrichova J, et al. Phenolic acid contents of kale (*Brassica oleraceae* L. var. acephala DC.) extracts and their antioxidant and antibacterial activities. Food Chemistry. 2008;**107**(1):19-25

[51] Dhanavade MJ, Jalkute CB, Ghosh JS, Sonawane KD. Study antimicrobial activity of lemon (*Citrus lemon* L.) peel extract. British Journal of Pharmacology and Toxicology. 2011;**2**(3):119-122

[52] Hayek SA, Gyawali R, Ibrahim SA. Antimicrobial natural products. In: Méndez-Vilas A, editor. Microbial Pathogens and Strategies for Combating Them: Science, Technology and Education. Vol. 2. USA: Formatex Research Center; 2013. pp. 910-921

[53] Rasooli I, Rezaei MB, Allameh A. Growth inhibition and morphological alterations of *Aspergillus niger* by essential oils from *Thymus eriocalyx* and *Thymus x-porlock*. Food Control. 2006; **17**(5):359-364

[54] Al-Habib A, Al-Saleh E, Safer A-M, Afzal M. Bactericidal effect of grape seed extract on methicillin-resistant *Staphylococcus aureus* (MRSA). The Journal of Toxicological Sciences. 2010; **35**(3):357-364

[55] Wu VC-H, Qiu X, Bushway A, Harper L. Antibacterial effects of American cranberry (*Vaccinium macrocarpon*) concentrate on foodborne pathogens. LWT-Food Science and Technology. 2008;**41**(10): 1834-1841

[56] Raybaudi-Massilia RM, Mosqueda-Melgar J, Martin-Belloso O. Antimicrobial activity of essential oils on *Salmonella enteritidis*, *Escherichia coli*, and *Listeria innocua* in fruit juices. Journal of Food Protection. 2006;**69**(7): 1579-1586

[57] Belguith H, Kthiri F, Ben Ammar A, Jaafoura H, Hamida JB, Landoulsi A. Morphological and biochemical changes of *Salmonella hadar* exposed to aqueous garlic extract. International Journal of Morphology. 2009;**27**(3)

[58] Stark J. Natamycin: An effective fungicide for food and beverages. In: Roller S, editor. Natrural Antimicrobials for the Minimal Processing of Foods. Cambridge: Woodhead Publishing Ltd; 2003

[59] Tsai G-J, Wu Z-Y, Wen-Huey S. Antibacterial activity of a chitooligosaccharide mixture prepared by cellulase digestion of shrimp chitosan and its application to milk preservation. Journal of Food Protection. 2000;**63**(6): 747-752

[60] No HK, Na YP, Lee SH, Meyers SP. Antibacterial activity of chitosans and chitosan oligomers with different molecular weights. International Journal of Food Microbiology. 2002;**74**(1–2): 65-72

[61] Katikou P, Ambrosiadis I, Georgantelis D, Koidis P, Georgakis SA. Effect of Lactobacillus-protective cultures with bacteriocin-like inhibitory substances' producing ability on microbiological, chemical and sensory

changes during storage of refrigerated vacuum-packaged sliced beef. Journal of Applied Microbiology. 2005;**99**(6): 1303-1313

[62] Castellano P, González C, Carduza F, Vignolo G. Protective action of *Lactobacillus curvatus* CRL705 on vacuum-packaged raw beef. Effect on sensory and structural characteristics. Meat Science. 2010;**85**(3):394-401

[63] Castellano P, Belfiore C, Vignolo G. Combination of bioprotective cultures with EDTA to reduce *Escherichia coli* O157: H7 in frozen ground-beef patties. Food Control. 2011;**22**(8):1461-1465

[64] Brillet A, Pilet M-F, Prevost H, Cardinal M, Leroi F. Effect of inoculation of *Carnobacterium divergens* V41, a biopreservative strain against *Listeria monocytogenes* risk, on the microbiological, chemical and sensory quality of cold-smoked salmon. International Journal of Food Microbiology. 2005;**104**(3):309-324

[65] Yang E, Fan L, Jiang Y, Doucette C, Fillmore S. Antimicrobial activity of bacteriocin-producing lactic acid bacteria isolated from cheeses and yogurts. AMB Express. 2012;**2**(1):48

[66] Barefoot SF, Klaenhammer TR. Detection and activity of lactacin B, a bacteriocin produced by *Lactobacillus acidophilus*. Applied and Environmental Microbiology. 1983;**45**(6):1808-1815

[67] Muriana PM, Klaenhammer TR. Purification and partial characterization of lactacin F, a bacteriocin produced by *Lactobacillus acidophilus* 11088. Applied and Environmental Microbiology. 1991; **57**(1):114-121

[68] Hurst A. Nisin. In: Advances in Applied Microbiology. Vol. 27. Netherlands: Academic Press; 1981. pp. 85-123

[69] McAuliffe O, Ryan MP, Paul Ross R, Hill C, Breeuwer P, Abee T. Lacticin 3147, a broad-spectrum bacteriocin which selectively dissipates the membrane potential. Applied and Environmental Microbiology. 1998; **64**(2):439-445

Chapter 3

Using Native Plants of the Northeast of Mexico for Developing Active Antimicrobial Food Packaging Films

Cecilia Rojas de Gante, Judith A. Rocha and Carlos P. Sáenz Collins

Abstract

The development of active food packaging is addressed using polyolefins such as LDPE and PVOH, as well as biopolymers from flour (sorghum and corn) and by-products of the food industry. Bacteriocins (nisin, natamycin), plant extracts such as oregano and thyme, as well as native plants of the northeast region of Mexico (*Larrea tridentata*, *Schinus molle*, *Cordia boissieri*, *Leucophyllum frutescens*), and essential oils of oregano and thyme as antimicrobial agents have been studied. The effect exerted by the process of incorporation of the antimicrobial agent (casting, extrusion) on the barrier and mechanical properties of the package as well as the antimicrobial activity of the containers (broad spectrum or selective activity) has been observed and the establishment of methods for their traceability.

Keywords: sorghum, maize, flour, nisin, thyme, oregano, *Larrea tridentata*, *Schinus molle*, *Cordia boissieri*, *Leucophyllum frutescens*, *Listeria monocytogenes*, *Staphylococcus aureus*

1. Introduction

Since the last decade and a half (2000 to date), the main forces that have unleashed the greatest developments in the packaging of food are the great concern of society for the care of their integral health including its nutritional status through foods with less or no presence of additives but in convenient presentations that facilitate their preparation, heating, and intake as well as foods with therapeutic action. A consumer who is very concerned about the safety of food, where food packaging and storage systems do not represent or have physical, biological, or even toxicological risks, nor for the protection of the environment.

All of the previous demand constantly forces the change on the nature of the food packaging and consequently on the materials of which it is composed [1]. Therefore, new materials are being developed to comply with the above. First, packages that contain in their formulation substances that migrate from the container to the food exert a positive action avoiding deterioration reactions likewise increase the sensory quality through the positive migration of substances or have a therapeutic effect. In this category are the so-called active packaging [1]. Second, in relation to the protection of the environment: the development of biodegradable packaging using, for example, biomaterials obtained from agri-food sources [1].

An active packaging is defined as the one that produces a change in the state of the packaged food to prolong its shelf life, improve its safety and quality, and provide a barrier between the food and its environment [1]. The mechanisms of action in active packages can be acting as emitting systems or as sequestering systems for substances. In the emitting systems, compounds or additives generally recognized as safe (GRAS), such as antioxidants and antimicrobial agents, are released into the food through the walls of the package. Sequestering systems remove undesirable compounds such as oxygen, H_2O, ethylene, CO_2, and impurities, among others [2]. Great diversity of active packaging is being developed in order to control the emission or absorption of substances and thus modify the environment of the product or directly the product. Thus, active packaging has substances or systems that absorb oxygen, ethylene, CO_2 and humidity; others absorb or release desired aromas [2–4]. Other active packages contain active enzyme systems and antimicrobial substances or systems. All these active containers seek the elimination of microbial growth, the extension of the useful life, and/or the increase of organoleptic qualities of the product [5].

The proposal of our line of research is based on obtaining a series of products (active antimicrobial and active biodegradable packages according to a defined food or conservation need), as well as the processes for their elaboration. Most developments use materials obtained only from starches or proteins. With our development, a single product has a biopolymer matrix that includes both biopolymers (starches and proteins) in a single stage. By starting from a matrix that includes both biopolymers (starches and proteins and sometimes antimicrobials or antioxidants), unit operations are eliminated, which reduces costs of equipment and energy, consequently operating costs. The technological impact of the developments of the research line will be reflected in the conservation of food (fresh or dehydrated) through the use of antimicrobial/antioxidant active packaging that contribute to preserve the environment when they are discarded since they are potentially biodegradable.

From the scientific point of view, this solves a couple of problems at the same time, the first concerning the toxicological risk of the abuse of additives in the formulation and conservation of food and the second discarding the ecological and environmental problems generated by food packaging. Our developments will have, on the one hand, low environmental impact due to the development of biodegradable products from nature-friendly processes. On the other hand, they will have a high economic impact since currently in the country there are no companies dedicated to the development of biopolymer containers, creation of own technologies, and high added value to products of low commercial value.

2. Antimicrobial active packaging developed at the Tecnológico de Monterrey

2.1 Biopolymer active packaging

Our first works focused on the use of starches from several varieties of sorghum (high-production cereal in northeast of Mexico) whose different proportion in amylose and amylopectin plays an important role in the water vapor barrier of the containers reinforcing them with prolamines (kafirin and zein) to increase their impermeability [6] and use of antifungal agents such as the sorbates and benzoates of Na and K. The inclusion of broad-spectrum antimicrobial additives in plastic polymers and/or biopolymers through the proprietary technology generated at the Tecnológico de Monterrey, for example, enabled active packaging to be obtained on a laboratory scale that reduced biological risks by manual or semi-manual packaging (risks of contamination with pathogens such as *Listeria monocytogenes* and *E. coli* O157: H7) [7–9]. On the other hand, there is great interest in the development and research of biopolymers obtained from agricultural sources. The matrices most commonly used to obtain this type of biopolymers are starch, proteins, and other polysaccharides. Some examples are corn zein, gluten and wheat gliadin, soy proteins, sorghum kafirin, cactus mucilage, and different types of starch (corn, potato, banana, tapioca, pea, waxy starch, and high amylose content, among others) [10–13]. In works carried out by our research group, it has been shown that it is possible to incorporate natural antimicrobial agents into films that could be used as active packaging. For example, Schause succeeded in establishing both the dry extraction conditions of starches and proteins from cereals such as sorghum (*Sorghum bicolor* Moench) as well as the casting process to obtain a film from sorghum flour and incorporate nisin as an antimicrobial active compound [8]. Nisin is a bacteriocin produced by some strains of *Lactococcus lactis* and *Streptococcus lactis* that has a broad antimicrobial power against Gram-positive bacteria. Nisin and lysozyme are used as a food preservative in dairy products as an inhibitor of *Clostridium tyrobutyricum*, *Clostridium butyricum*, *Clostridium saccharobutyricum* (causes swelling in cheese production), and pathogens like *Clostridium botulinum*, *Clostridium sporogenes* (which is used as a surrogate for *C. botulinum*), and *L. monocytogenes* [14]. The bactericidal action of nisin occurs in the cytoplasmic membrane, causing cell damage due to proton loss and damage to the integrity of the cell membrane [14]. Gram-negative bacteria have an outer membrane that protects the cytoplasmic membrane, so the bactericidal action of nisin is limited and the development of Gram-negative bacteria such as *E. coli* O157: H7 and *Salmonella* would not be inhibited.

Subsequently, Ríos-Licea conducted a search of natural substances of broad spectrum, so he analyzed the antimicrobial activity of aqueous extracts of known plants. Ríos-Licea also succeeded in developing antimicrobial films by incorporating natural extracts of garlic and oregano into the same biopolymer matrix of sorghum flour using the method established by Schause [15]. However, it was necessary to incorporate high concentrations of natural extracts, due to the low potency of the antimicrobial activity of the commercial product tested.

Tinoco-Pérez studied a variety of corn rich in anthocyanins (blue corn) by applying the process of dry milling and establishing the process to obtain active films in antioxidants (anthocyanins) from flour of this cereal [16]. Two biopolymers present in corn with a filmogenic capacity are starch and zein, the first being the most abundant in this grain [16]. There are a significant amount of reports published on films made from corn starch and zein; the effect of different additives, copolymers, and processes on the performance of films for different applications has been evaluated. In 2009, Mexico produced 29.4 million tons of corn using 38.5% of its total cultivated area. The production of this grain has shown an increase in its average annual growth rate of 2.1% in the period from 1994 to 2008. Of total corn production in 2008, 92% was white corn, 7% was blue corn, and 1% was of other varieties. Basically, white corn is destined for national consumption, yellow for export, and the rest of the varieties are commonly produced for self-consumption of rural populations. Among the 1% of the varieties not defined is the blue corn (*Zea mays* amylacea) [17, 18]. Blue corn (*Zea mays* amylacea) is a type of corn rich in anthocyanins (responsible for its pigmentation) and floury endosperm. It is cultivated in areas of dry climate and demands minimal care. Despite its nutraceutical potential, blue corn is only produced by rural communities for self-consumption due to its devalued commercial value, since the urbanized areas consume mainly white and yellow corn products. Among the few current uses of blue corn is the extraction of anthocyanins for use as natural food coloring and antioxidants [16, 19].

Among the processes studied to obtain films from corn fractions are casting, different types of extrusion (double screw/flat die, single screw/flat die, and extrusion/calendering, among others), stretching of zein resins, and pressing by heat [10, 20–22]. The effects of various additives and chemical treatments, for example, plasticizers, hydrophobic agents, copolymers, and the use of chemically modified starches on the structural, molecular, thermal, mechanical, and barrier performance characteristics, have been studied extensively [22–25].

In the case of sorghum, the cultivation of this cereal is less demanding in agronomic terms than corn (water and nutrients) [26, 27]. Sorghum is the fifth most important grain in the world, being the United States the country with the highest production in the world, followed by India and Nigeria. For the year 2010, Mexico contributed with 10.5% of the total world production, equivalent to 6,250,000 metric tons [15, 16]. In Mexico, sorghum is the second most important grain in production after corn; during the period 1996–2006, sorghum production contributed with 22% of the total production of cereals [26].

In Mexico, this cereal is destined mainly for livestock feed and secondarily for human food and obtaining inputs such as starch, alcohol, glucose, acetone, and butanol. One of the great advantages of sorghum is that it has the capacity to adapt to arid and semiarid climatic conditions and to be resistant to drought for long periods [26]. In previous works, it was able to demonstrate that antimicrobial active films can be obtained from corn and sorghum flour [8, 15, 16].

The biopolymers obtained in this way through a technique and process patented by Tecnológico de Monterrey as PCT [28] have the advantage of being biodegradable because their chemical structure is primarily based on proteins and starches. Additionally, they have the possibility of forming films with plasticity (custom flexibility) and of being formulated also tailored to the requirements of the product to be packaged. Additionally, they can be heat sealed to form bags of different dimensions or not to be sealed and act as "active" pads or pads in combination with other packaging. In addition to the advantages in terms of sustainability, the interest in using these sources to produce biopolymers lies in adding value to agricultural products [8, 29].

It is important to note that for any application of the said technology, it will be necessary to make an adaptation of the formulations and the process to satisfy the specific protection requirements for each food to be packaged. For what it is proposed to demonstrate in this work, the film-like packages obtained by adapting the formulations and process of the said published patent work to preserve and keep refrigerated for 30–45 days a commercial presentation in slices of semi-matured cheese [30].

The biopolymeric antimicrobial films described in WO2010/024657 A1 from cereals are limited to the packaging of dry foods or as pads for adsorption of exudates and emission of antimicrobial agents for fresh meat and cheese products [28]. Because of its sensitivity to water and low mechanical resistance to contain products with intermediate moisture, the biopolymeric matrix was reformulated to improve both parameters [30]. The results of refrigerated shelf stability of the cheese in terms of the control capacity exercised by the antimicrobials used in this study (nisin and natamycin) through the active packaging against fungi and yeast were effective throughout storage compared to vacuum packaging (control). The results of the microbial kinetics throughout the refrigerated storage for the fungi and yeast count showed the effectiveness of the active packaging. The development of fungi and yeasts remained controlled, showing the effectiveness of this emerging food preservation technology [30].

The plasticizing effects of two different polyols (glycerol and sorbitol) on the mechanical, thermal, and microstructural properties of flour films were studied by Valderrama and Rojas, and the results showed that films plasticized with sorbitol had better mechanical properties and less affinity for water than those plasticized with glycerol. The attenuated total reflectance-Fourier-transform infrared (ATR-FTIR) spectra of blue corn flour plasticizer with sorbitol showed the presence of the additional band at 1745 cm^{-1} characteristic of the carbonyl peak, which confirms the chemical linkages between sorbitol and a polymeric matrix. The effect of the plasticizer on the glass transition temperature (Tg) showed that Tg decreased as the plasticizer content increased. Plasticized glycerol films showed lower Tg values than those with sorbitol. Observations by scanning electron microscopy (SEM) showed that it was necessary to add plasticizer to maintain film integrity. The sorbitol-plasticized flour films revealed better adhesion between phases, and these films showed a compact structure [31].

Finally, bioplastics were produced through thermoplastic processing using different cereals derived raw materials, namely, blue maize flour (BM), white sorghum flour (WS), maize starch, and the maize prolamin (zein). The overall performance of the bioplastics was investigated emphasizing on the study of the effect of different process strategies on the compatibilization of the starch and prolamin using mixtures of urea and formamide (UF) and maleated starch (MS) as compatibilizing agents [32, 33]. Results suggest that two competing phenomena, thermoplasticization and degradation, occurred simultaneously during the thermoplastic process. Fourier-transform infrared (FTIR) spectroscopy analysis evidenced the chemical changes induced by these phenomena. Moreover, chemical modification had also a major effect on the properties of the produced materials. WS films made with chemically modified flour increased their tensile strength in 29%, as compared to their native counterparts. Thermogravimetric analysis and FTIR analysis showed that the chemical interaction between starch and zein occurred more extensively in films made with formamide than those made with maleated starch [32, 33].

2.2 Plastic active packaging

In Valderrama's work, natural aqueous extracts are exchanged for essential oils because they have a higher concentration of antimicrobial active substances. It analyzed essential oils of oregano, thyme, tea tree, and mint, which have greater antimicrobial activity than the natural extracts used by Ríos-Licea [15]. In particular, the effect of incorporating two essential oils such as oregano (*Origanum vulgare*) and thyme (*Thymus vulgaris*) on polyolefin materials such as low-density polyethylene (LDPE) and polypropylene (PP) was studied.

The mechanical, barrier, and antimicrobial properties of the packaging were evaluated against *Salmonella typhimurium*, *Listeria monocytogenes*, and *Escherichia coli* O157:H7. The results demonstrate that films developed by extrusion incorporating 4% (w/w) of essential oils had a higher inhibitory effect than those obtained using the ionizing treatment. The packaging developed by extrusion containing 1% (w/w) showed a positive inhibitory effect, while those obtained by the ionizing treatment had no inhibitory effect against any of the test microorganisms. The incorporation of essential oils on the LDPE films generated a plasticizer effect, whereas the ones obtained by means of ionizing treatment did significantly affect the barrier properties of the films Valderrama and Rojas [9].

A simple and rapid Fourier-transform infrared (FTIR) spectroscopy method was developed by Valderrama and Rojas to determine the main essential oil components (carvacrol, thymol, and p-cymene) in the antimicrobial LDPE films incorporated with oregano (*Origanum vulgare*) and thyme (*Thymus vulgaris*) essential oils. The ATR-FTIR spectroscopy with chemometrics, using the PLS-first derivative spectra, could predict the active compounds content accurate to an r2 >0.99 and a standard error of prediction (SEP) of <0.7. The developed method was successfully applied to predict the concentration of active compounds: carvacrol, thymol, and p-cymene in oregano and thyme essential oils with results compared to those of the GC-MS method. The described nondestructive method can be applied to make the traceability of active compounds of essential oils in antimicrobial food packaging [34].

The work of Rocha is described below, who worked with the same essential oils of oregano and thyme that Valderrama used to obtain active plastic containers. This was due to the fact that they presented greater antimicrobial activity than the aqueous extracts of oregano and garlic from previous studies in our research group [9, 15]. It also proposed the use of a polymeric film for the preparation of the active container with essential oils, in order to present an alternative to vacuum cheese packaging. For this project, polyvinyl alcohol (PVOH) has been chosen for the preparation of the packaging due to its unique characteristics: permeability, biodegradability, and its facility to form films by the casting method. The purpose of this work is to propose an alternative, a packaging that is not dependent on complex plastic structures that requires vacuum packaging for provide the high barrier. The main challenge of the present project is the incorporation of essential oils that are lipophilic to a hydrophilic PVOH matrix, which is why it was suggested encapsulating them in cyclodextrins.

3. Control of the development of *Listeria monocytogenes* in fresh cheese during shelf life at refrigeration by means of an antimicrobial PVOH film (pad) with microcapsules of active compounds of oregano and thyme

The presence of *Listeria* spp. has been found in cheeses from developed countries such as the United States, Sweden, France, Germany, Italy, Brazil, and Japan. Hence, there is an urgent need to find alternative conservation systems, which allow to contribute to the inhibition of this type of pathogen. Listeriosis infections represent only 0.02% of cases of diseases in the USA; however, this bacterium is responsible for 25% of deaths in outbreaks related to food [35, 36]. Especially worrisome is the fact that it can survive pasteurization and be able to develop even in refrigeration temperatures. Hence, the importance of finding new technologies for their control and/or elimination, in particular, considering that the use of antimicrobial compounds in dairy products is restricted, that there is great interest in using natural compounds for this purpose but, above all, that these substances are added to the containers and not to the food, which can be achieved through the active packaging, is the objective of the present study. The development of *L. monocytogenes* has a particular health interest, because it is responsible for a fifth of the deaths related to foodborne diseases, especially considering that it survives the pasteurization process and develops even in refrigeration. It is important to highlight the tendency to decrease and, in some cases, eliminate preservatives in food. In dairy products, the direct use of antimicrobial agents is specifically forbidden, so the use of natural additives is becoming an alternative. If these are combined with the primary function of packaging to maintain sanitary safety and minimize the toxicological impacts of food, we are getting an active packaging. An active container that inhibits its development in fresh cheese during its storage in refrigeration can help to reduce the incidence of outbreaks and deaths due to this bacterium. The main goal was to develop an active packaging system that allows to control the development of pathogenic bacteria, in particular *Listeria monocytogenes* in refrigerated fresh cheeses, using natural antibacterial agents. As specific objectives: select and establish the conditions of incorporation of essential oils in a hydrophilic polymer, polyvinyl alcohol (PVOH), studying three methods of incorporation and formation of films; determine the antimicrobial activity of the films obtained against *Salmonella typhimurium*, *Listeria monocytogenes*, and *Escherichia coli* O157: H7 as target microorganisms; and, finally, check the effectiveness of the film and packaging system in the inhibition of the development of *L. monocytogenes* in fresh goat cheese, during 29 days of refrigerated storage.

3.1 Methods

3.1.1 Selection of substances, materials, microorganisms, and cheese

The selected essential oils were oregano (OEO) and thyme (TEO) (Primavera Life) for their potent antimicrobial activity and their availability in the national market. The antimicrobial activity of these inclusion complexes such as films using *Salmonella typhimurium*, *Listeria monocytogenes*, and *Escherichia coli* O157:H7 as target microorganisms was determined. Polyvinyl alcohol (PVOH) soluble in hot water, 87–90% hydrolyzed, with a molecular weight of 30,000–70,000 (Sigma-Aldrich), and glycerol (DEQ) were used for the production of active film. To obtain the inclusion complexes of the essential oils, crystalline α-cyclodextrin and β-cyclodextrin (Sigma-Aldrich) were used. The plastic films for the cheese packaging were LDPE film made by extrusion by Valderrama [9] and multilayer film Zublon® 5CR (Zubex Industrial S.A. de C.V.). For the activation of the microorganisms, the following selective broths were used: UVM-modified Listeria Enrichment Broth for *L. monocytogenes* (Becton Dickinson, DIFCO, México), Brilliant green bile lactose broth (BRILA broth) for *E.coli* O157: H7 (Merck KGaA, Germany), and Brain Heart Infusion broth (BHI broth) for *S. typhimurium* (Merck KGaA, Germany). For the plate count and antimicrobial activity tests, the following were used: Oxford Agar for *L. monocytogenes* (Becton Dickinson, DIFCO, México), SS agar for *Salmonella* and *Shigella* (Merck KGaA, Germany), Modified EC Broth and Bacto Agar for *E. coli* (Becton Dickinson, DIFCO, México). Oxford Agar with Oxford selective supplement (Becton Dickinson, DIFCO, México) was used for the counting of *L. monocytogenes* in the fresh cheese packaged experiment. For the goat cheese, fresh goat cheese, CAPRICO brand Cabrero cheese, was obtained in 400 g presentations directly with the company CAPRICO (manufacturing lot JL09210PN) located in Linares, N.L.

3.1.2 Process for developing PVOH films with active microcapsules of essential oils

The PVOH films were elaborated adapting the method used by Schause [8] and Ríos-Licea [15], previously studying three methods of incorporation of the essential oils in it: dispersion, emulsification, and formation of inclusion complexes with α and β cyclodextrins (CD) and the following variables: amount of PVOH, type and amount of cyclodextrin, coprecipitation strategy, solvent (water, ethanol), and concentration of EO. The encapsulation with β-CD is being the one selected for the incorporation of EO in the PVOH film. A PVOH film without inclusion complex was made as a control. With the resulting films, pads of 8 × 4 cm were made to be used in the active packaging system.

3.1.3 Thermal stability of essential oils and confirmation of inclusion complex formation by differential thermal analysis (DTA)

In order to determine the degradation temperature of the essential oils and establish if these would be affected during the film making process, the thermal stability of the same and their active compounds were evaluated. Firstly, a thermal evaluation of the essential oils of oregano and thyme was carried out, as well as its main active components with carvacrol, thymol, and p-cymene standards. Next, the β-CD and the inclusion complexes of OEO and TEO to confirm the formation of such complexes and not only a physical mixture. Finally, a thermal evaluation of the PVOH films with the inclusion complexes of CD:EO of oregano and thyme was made to determine the optimal storage temperature of the active films. The thermal evaluation was performed with a home DTA validated by Martínez and collaborators [37]. For each substance, at least two runs of food matrix were performed to verify the repeatability of the analysis.

3.1.4 Microbiological evaluation and disk diffusion method

To determine the antimicrobial activity of PVOH films, the disk diffusion method was applied (Kirby-Bauer method). After preparing and inoculating the agar with 10^6 CFU of each microorganism, samples of the films were cut in the form of 6 mm diameter disks and deposited on the agar, evaluating both the rough and smooth side of the films [7, 38, 39]. After 24 hours of incubation at 37 ± 1°C in inverted position, the inhibition halo was measured with a digital micrometer (Mitutoyo Digimatic 2,931,051 m, 0.001 mm sensitivity).

3.1.5 Control study of *L. monocytogenes* in fresh goat cheese using an active packaging system

The packaging system consisted of a pad of PVOH with EO microcapsules of oregano and thyme in a LDPE bag. First, 7 × 7 cm bags with LDPE film of 0.023 ± 0.003 mm thickness obtained by extrusion by Valderrama [9] were made, which were obtained by sealing two films on three sides with a vacuum packing machine Torrey brand. In the same way, bags were obtained with the multilayer film (Zublon® 5CR from Zubex Industrial). Second, in aseptic conditions, portions of cheese of 3 cm × 3 cm and 10 ± 0.5 g of weight were cut and exposed to UV treatment for 15 min on each side, a methodology adapted from Suppakul [40] for the purpose to reduce the interference of microorganisms typical of cheese in the study. Then, the samples were packed in the bags of the four treatments to be analyzed and inoculated with 100 mL of *Listeria monocytogenes* at a concentration of 5 × 10^3 CFU/mL. Finally, the bags were heat sealed in a packaging machine (TORREY) and stored in a refrigerator (Torrey Model VRD42) at 4 ± 1°C for up to 29 days.

The four treatments evaluated were (1) multilayer bag for vacuum packaging as control, (2) LDPE bag with PVOH "pad" without essential oils, (3) LDPE bag with PVOH "pad" with inclusion complex of β-CD:OEO, essential oil at a concentration of 25% in the film, and (4) LDPE bag with PVOH "pad" with inclusion complex of β-CD:TEO, essential oil at a concentration of 25% in the film.

The inhibition kinetics of *L. monocytogenes* was determined in the cheese samples packaged at 0, 1, 3, 5, 7, 15, 22, 26, and 29 days at refrigerated conditions. The analysis of the microbial count proceeded according to NOM110-SSA1-1994, making decimal dilutions and plate count [41]. The LabVIEW software for differential thermal analysis was used.

3.2 Results

3.2.1 PVOH films process with microcapsules of essential oils of oregano and thyme

It was possible to produce PVOH films with the inclusion complexes of oregano and thyme in all the experimental conditions. Films with 1, 4, and 15% EO were prepared with molar ratio 1:10, which they are shown in **Figure 1**. Films made with 1% EO were those most similar to the PVOH control film. Continuous, elastic, and transparent films were obtained. The higher the concentration of the essential oil in the film, the more presence of the inclusion complex affects the transparency of the film, with the PVOH matrix being observed as white, as can be seen in the film at 15% EO (**Figure 1**). It should be noted, however, that although the inclusion complex is observed in the film, no migration of this or the essential oil to the touch is perceived, which is why it has been well incorporated into the PVOH matrix. The films also presented less transparency when approaching the β-CD:EO ratio at 1:1

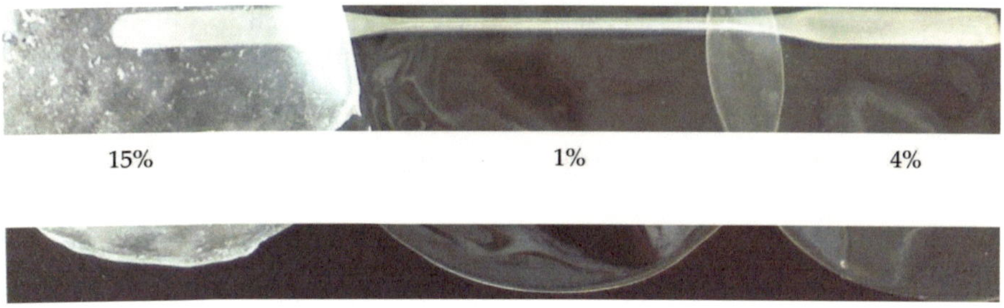

Figure 1.
Appearance of PVOH films with different concentrations of inclusion complex. Films elaborated at concentrations of 1, 4, and 15% of EO by process A (molar ratio β-CD: AO 1:10).

molar proportions; this is because a greater amount of inclusion complex tends to saturate the film. The films whose inclusion complex was dissolved in 30% ethanol also showed greater transparency than those in which it was prepared in water; this is because the inclusion complex in the 30% ethanol solution was better solubilized.

3.2.2 Thermal stability of essential oils and confirmation of inclusion complex formation by DTA

Firstly, the thermal stability of β-cyclodextrin and the essential oils of oregano and thyme, as well as its components (carvacrol, thymol, and p-cymene), was evaluated to confirm the formation of inclusion complexes. The thermograms of the carvacrol, thymol, and p-cymene standards are shown in **Figure 2** and **3**. Here it is shown that these three components are stable up to a temperature of 182°C, which refers to the boiling temperature of the p-cymene. The melting point of thymol shown in **Figure 2** is in agreement with that obtained by Ponce, which reports the melting point of thymol at 50°C [42]. The boiling point of p-cymene matches with the one reported by the supplier (178–180°C Sigma-Aldrich). Carvacrol was analyzed by broadening the study temperatures, as shown in **Figure 3**. This compound has an interesting behavior, since it has a crystallization temperature of −20°C followed by a melting point of 2°C and a point of boiling of 240° C. Sigma-Aldrich reports its melting point at 3–4°C and its boiling point at 236–237°C, which also coincides with that reported by Dahmane, which reports the boiling point of carvacrol at 237.7°C [43]. The closeness of the crystallization and fusion transitions does not allow the existence of a solid state of this intermediate substance at the reported temperatures. A similar behavior is reported by Ponce for cinnamaldehyde [42]. According to the obtained in **Figure 5**, it was successful to form an inclusion complex, since otherwise the signal of the boiling point would have been shown at 214°C of the essential oils (**Figure 4**).

The thermogram obtained by DTA of the β-CD:EO inclusion complexes of oregano and thyme (**Figure 5**) shows that they are stable at temperatures below 115°C, so there is no risk of degradation of the active compounds if the inclusion complex dissolves PVOH in situ in a solution with inclusion complex at 8°C (process B of PVOH film making with inclusion complexes). **Figure 6** shows the thermogram of the PVOH films with the inclusion complexes of oregano and thyme. The film made with essential oil of thyme had a little moisture on its surface, so we can see a couple of peaks at 0 and 100°C corresponding to the melting and boiling point of water, respectively. PVOH control films and those with inclusion complexes of essential oil of oregano and thyme are stable up to a temperature of 110°C, which indicates that they can be stored in shelves at room temperature without problem.

The PVOH control film has a peak at 150°C, which refers to the point of fusion of unplasticized PVOH. The last peak corresponds to the degradation of PVOH at 230°C, which is supported by Holland and Hay [44].

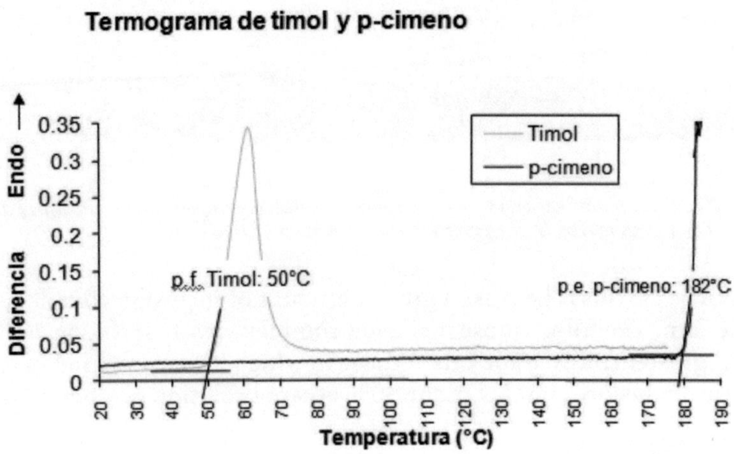

Figure 2.
Thermogram of thymol and p-cymene.

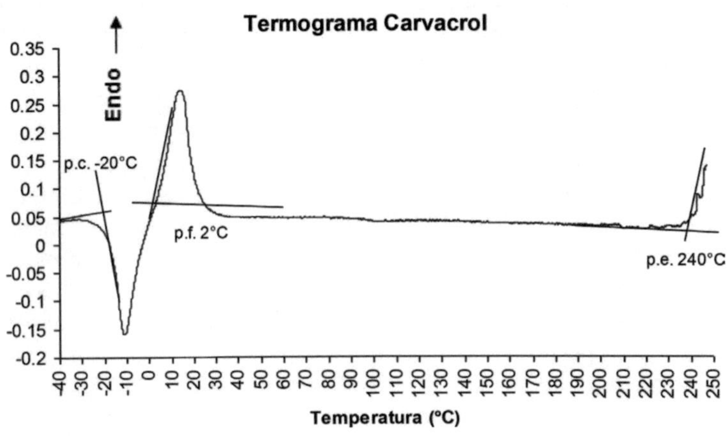

Figure 3.
Carvacrol thermogram.

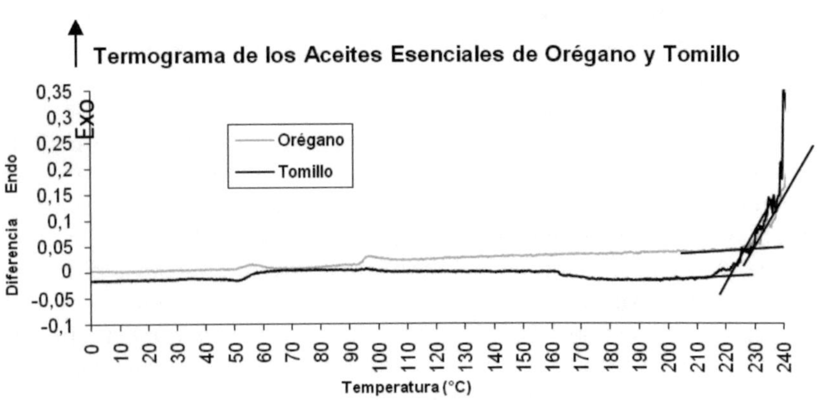

Figure 4.
Thermogram of thyme and oregano essential oils.

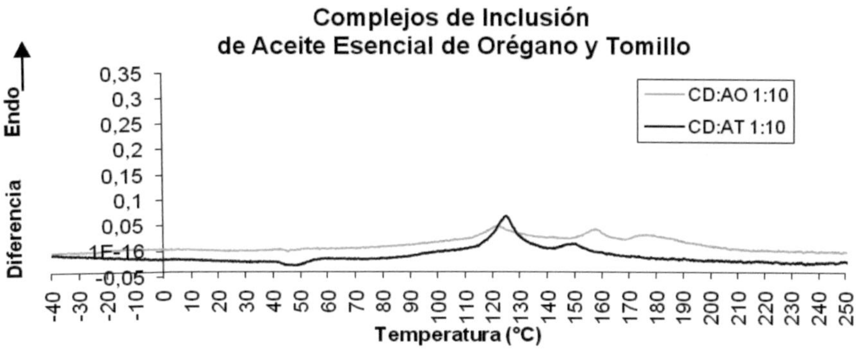

Figure 5.
Thermogram of the inclusion complexes of OEO and TEO with β–CD.

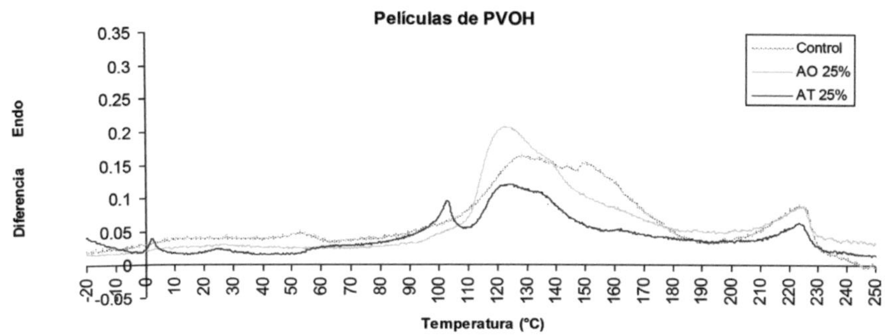

Figure 6.
Thermogram of PVOH films with inclusion complexes of OEO and TEO.

3.2.3 Antimicrobial activity of the active films in vitro against L. monocytogenes, S. typhimurium, and E. coli O157: H7

The films made with a concentration of 25% essential oil of oregano and thyme presented broad-spectrum antimicrobial activity by inhibiting the growth against the Gram-positive and Gram-negative microorganisms evaluated. The antimicrobial activity and the inhibition halo against *E. coli* O157: H7, *L. monocytogenes*, and *S. typhimurium* is shown in **Figure 7**. In this test the antimicrobial activity of both films was very similar against *E. coli* O157: H7 and *S. typhimurium*. The opposite occurred against *L. monocytogenes*, where the films with 25% of TEO showed higher antimicrobial activity than the films with 25% of OEO. The halos of inhibition against *E. coli* O157: H7 and *S. typhimurium* shown in **Figure 7(A)** and **(C)** suggest that the rough side of the film shows a slightly higher antimicrobial activity against microorganisms, a capacity that was confirmed in the analysis against *L. monocytogenes* (**Figure 7(B)**). The treatment of the film with the highest antimicrobial activity was that elaborated at 25% of essential oil, with the inclusion complex in molar ratio β-CD:EO 1:10 and evaluated by its rough side. In experimental designs not reported in this work, we could verify that both, the concentration of the essential oil (1, 4, 8, 15%) and the molar ratio of the inclusion complex β-CD:EO (1:2 and 1:5), are factors that influence the antimicrobial activity, as well as the speed of diffusion of the antimicrobial through the walls of the microcapsule [45].

The antimicrobial activity of the films is mainly due to the phenol group of carvacrol and p-cymene. The concentration of these compounds in the essential oils of oregano and thyme used for the production of films is shown in **Table 1**. The

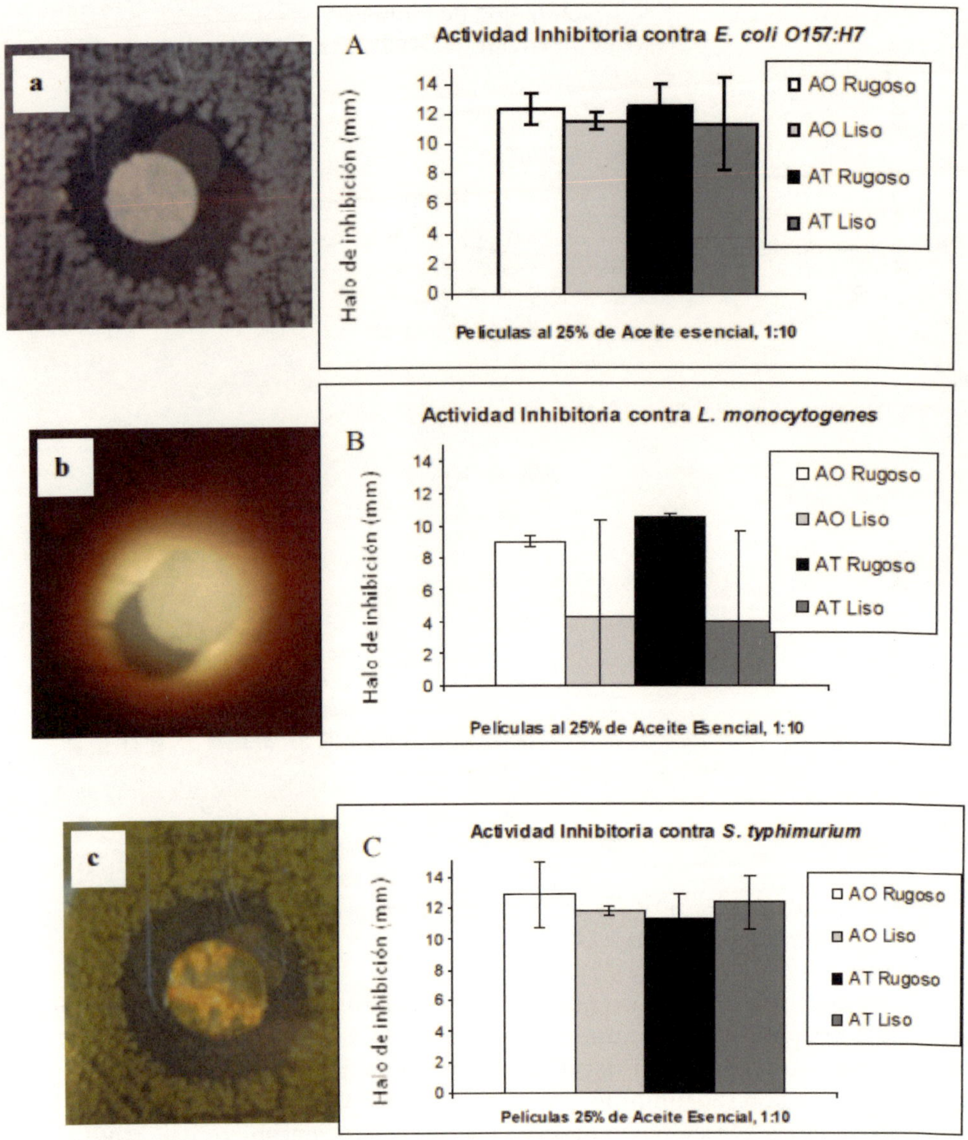

Películas de PVOH elaboradas con 25% de Aceite de Orégano (AO) y de Tomillo (AT) con relación molar 1:10 (β-CD:AE) frente a *E. coli* O157:H7 (A), *L. monocytogenes* (B) y *S. typhimurium* (C) y sus halos de inhibición (a),(b) y (c) respectivamente.

Figure 7.
Antimicrobial activity of PVOH fims with inclusion complexes against pathogenic bacteria. 7a against E. coli, 7b against L. monocytogenes, and 7c against S. typhimurium.

phenol group is essential for bacterial inhibition, since it destabilizes the cytoplasmic membrane and also functions as a proton exchanger which reduces the pH gradient in the membrane and causes cell collapse and death [46–48]. The destabilization of the membrane occurs because carvacrol and thymol have affinity for lipids and accumulates in the bilayer between fatty acid chains, which causes changes in the conformation of the membrane. This mechanism of action does not present p-cymene; however, it has been found to have a synergy with phenols, expanding the membrane and destabilizing it [46]. The position of the hydroxyl group in the phenolic compounds does not seem to influence the degree of antimicrobial activity so that the activity of carvacrol and thymol is similar.

Concentration*	Oregano Essential Oil	Thyme essential oil
Phenolic compounds (carvacrol and thymol)	77.7%	54.05%
Terpene compounds (p-cymene and other compounds)	20.07%	41.34%

*Concentrations determined from the GC analysis of the supplier´s quality certificates

Table 1.
Concentration of phenolic compounds in the OEO and TEO.

3.2.4 Analysis of the control of L. monocytogenes in fresh cheese packed during storage in a refrigerated rack

The antimicrobial activity of the PVOH films with inclusion complexes of oregano and thyme in a model with fresh cheese inoculated with *L. monocytogenes* and stored in a rack refrigerated at 4°C was evaluated. As seen in **Figure 8**, the pathogenic microorganism shows inhibition when it is packed with the films developed with the antimicrobial agents, since the fresh cheese develops fewer colonies than that packaged with PVOH control or with the multilayer film under vacuum. The concentration of *L. monocytogenes* gradually decreased in the cheeses packaged with the active pads as shown in **Figure 8**. After 15 days of storage, the cheese packed with the films with oregano and thyme no longer had a microbial count; this performance was better than in the cheeses packaged with the vacuum multilayer film (red line) that did present a microbial account. This fact would have been interpreted as that the films developed with inclusion complexes of oregano and thyme presented bactericidal activity against *L. monocytogenes* in cheese, in refrigerated shelf after 15 days of exposure. Unfortunately, the films do not have bactericidal activity since colonies were detected on days 22 and 26 of storage. For this reason, it is concluded that the active films have a bacteriostatic control against *L. monocytogenes*. It is also observed in **Figure 8**, that the vacuum multilayer film showed greater control of the microbial load of the inoculated cheese, than the package with PVOH film without essential oils. This is due to the fact that in vacuum packaging with multilayer film, the oxygen available in the head space is reduced, together with the gas impermeability of the film, preventing microorganisms from developing. *L. monocytogenes* in particular is

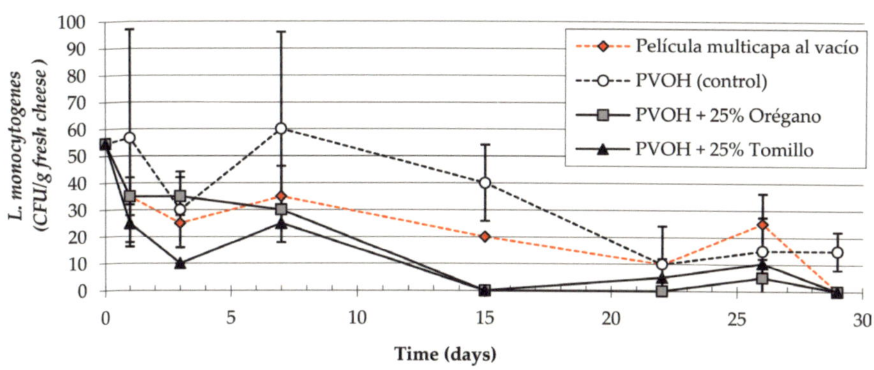

Figure 8.
Antimicrobial activity of PVOH films with inclusion complexes against fresh cheese inoculated with L. monocytogenes in refrigerated storage. PVOH films with 25% of OEO and TEO incorporated as inclusion complex. PVOH and multilayer vacuum packages were used as controls.

an aerobic bacterium, which is why the vacuum-packed product has control over its development during the time of storage.

3.3 Conclusions

Active PVOH films were obtained with essential oils of oregano and thyme, which showed broad-spectrum antibacterial activity by inhibiting pathogenic Gram-positive and Gram-negative bacteria specifically against *L. monocytogenes*, *E. coli* O157: H7, and *S. typhimurium*. The best conditions for the production of active films were 25% essential oil and elaboration of inclusion complex with a relation of 1:10 β-CD:EO. The active pad elaborated in the aforementioned conditions presented bacteriostatic activity against *L. monocytogenes* in cheese inoculated, packaged, and stored at 4°C for 29 days. The proposed packaging system ("pad" of the developed active film and a low-density polyethylene bag) can be an alternative to vacuum packaging using a multilayer film for cheeses. The experimental results showed that they provide a shelf life equivalent to vacuum packaging. In addition to the control of microbial activity, the proposed system is more accessible to small cheese producers as no special packaging technology is required other than a heat sealer machine. Likewise, the proposed packaging system can help reduce the incidence of outbreaks of diseases transmitted by foods contaminated with *Listeria monocytogenes*.

4. Antimicrobial agents from plants of the northeast of Mexico

As Mexico is a country that stands out for its floristic richness and taking into account the extensive knowledge of medicinal plants that since the pre-Columbian Era conserve Mexicans, mainly those of rural communities, it was natural that we were interested in the study of incorporation of some of them as active substances to be included in polymer matrices for food packaging.

4.1 *Larrea tridentata* plant as an alternative source for obtaining antimicrobial extracts

The flora of arid zones represents a great potential for the wealth based on its biological specialization, since it is the product of thousands of years of physiological adaptation for its survival [50]. The governor plant (*L. tridentata*) typically develops under conditions of these zones. The *Larrea* genus includes five species of evergreen shrubs distributed throughout the Americas; its name was given in honor of the Spanish cleric Juan Antonio Hernández Larrea who was dean of the Zaragoza Chapter and bishop of Valladolid. This plant is commonly known as the governor, due to its dominance in the large areas of the arid zones of northern Mexico, but it is also known as guamis, sonora, tasajo, jarilla, creosote, and hediondilla due to its characteristic smell, mainly after the rain. In the Seri language, it is called "haaxat," and in the English language it has the common names of "creosote bush" and "greasewood" [49, 50].

The governor plant has a wide range of adaptation in elevation since it is located in the Valley of Death in California located 86 m below sea level, to more than 2500 m in the sierras of northern Mexico. Its growth is good in dry plains and plateaus, also around hills and slopes, and in several types of soils except clayey, saline, or granitic [50]. The lifetime of this plant is negatively correlated with disturbance and soil compaction, being intolerant to soils with high phosphorus content [49]. In Mexico, the distribution of the governor plant is in part of the Sonoran Desert, which includes the states of Baja California, Baja California Sur and Sonora, and in the Chihuahuan Desert, which includes the states of Chihuahua, Durango, Coahuila, Nuevo León, Zacatecas, and San Luis Potosí [50]. The infusion of the whole *L. tridentata* plant especially of the branches is used in urinary tract disorders to undo the kidney stones. The firing of branches, root, and bark is used to treat discomforts such as kidney pain and bladder inflammation. The decoction of the leaves is suggested in vaginal washes in gynecological problems such as female sterility. The infusion of branches, root, and bark is used in baths to treat hemorrhoids, fever, malaria, pimples, bumps, good healing, and rheumatism. And the infusion of the leaves is used as a remedy for gallstones, rheumatism, dermatitis, hepatitis, antiseptic, gastric discomforts, venereal diseases, and tuberculosis, in addition to having antiamoebic activity [49, 51, 52].

Among the uses that the governor plant has traditionally had, it stands out in its use as an antioxidant that was given to it in the United States since 1943; although in the decade of the 1990s, it was suspended by the US Food and Drug Administration (FDA) due to the strong interaction of nordihydroguaiaretic acid (NDGA) comment on results that were not found in the extracts studied, with several enzymatic processes. NDGA inhibits enzymatic activity, in addition to inhibiting the signaling pathway of lipoxygenase in which arachidonic acid generates leukotrienes and other oxygenated products [53–55].

4.2 *Cordia boissieri* plant as an alternative source for obtaining antimicrobial extracts

The anacahuita plant (*Cordia boissieri*) is the official flower of the state of Nuevo León, México. The genus *Cordia* gets its name in honor of the sixteenth-century German botanist Valerius Cordus and the *boissieri* species gets its name in honor of the nineteenth-century French botanist Boissier [56]. This plant is commonly known by the names of anacahuita, Mexican olive, Texas olive, wild olive, trompillo, and rasca viejo [56]. *C. boissieri* is a shrub or small tree up to 5 m high, with ovate leaves, 15–20 cm long and velvety surface. The flowers are white, grouped from 5 to 8, with the yellow center, up to 45 mm in length. The fruit is ovoid from 25 to 30 mm, brownish-green to purple, fleshy, sweet, and contains 1–4 seeds [56]. This plant species is native to North America. It is mainly distributed in Mexico, in the states of Nuevo León, Coahuila, Tamaulipas, San Luis Potosí, and Veracruz, and in the State of Texas in the United States. There are reports that the fruits of the *C. boissieri* plant are used as a remedy for coughs and colds. Traditionally the leaves of the plant are used to treat rheumatism and bronchial problems. Also in traditional medicine, the flowers are used in the treatment of diseases of bacterial origin [51, 56, 57].

4.3 *Leucophyllum frutescens* plant as an alternative source for obtaining antimicrobial extracts

The ash plant (*Leucophyllum frutescens*) is an evergreen shrub. This plant is commonly known, in Mexico, with the name of ash and in the United States with the names of Texas ranger, Texas sage, silverleaf, and barometer bush, because the flowering is triggered by moisture [58]. It is a grey bush of 1.5–2 m in height. The silver-grey and green leaves are covered with silver hair. The violet to purple flowers are bell-shaped or funnel with five lobes and two lips and reach to measure 2.5 cm in length, which appear intermittently from spring to autumn. The fruit has the shape of a small capsule [58]. This plant is native to northern Mexico and the Southwestern United States. It is a species that is part of the medium and high bushes that develop preferably in *lomeríos* of capricious soils [59]. Reports were found that in traditional medicine the leaves of *Lecophyllum frutescens* are used in the treatment of diseases caused by bacteria [51]. No work has been found on the compounds present in *Leucophyllum frutescens* to which an antibacterial action against *S. aureus* can be attributed.

4.4 *Schinus molle* plant as an alternative source for obtaining antimicrobial extracts

The plant pirul (*Schinus molle*) is a perennial tree native to South America and naturalized in Mexico by Viceroy Antonio de Mendoza in the sixteenth century [60]. This plant is commonly known by the names of pirul in Mexico, aguaribay in Argentina, anacahuita in Uruguay, molle in Peru and, false pepper in Colombia [60]. It is a tree from 4 to 15 m high. The leaves are compound, alternate, 15–30 cm long, hung, with milky sap, and yellowish green. Its flowers are axillary panicles in the terminal leaves, 10–15 cm long, yellowish in color. The fruits are drupes in hanging clusters, each fruit 5–9 mm in diameter, pink or red [60]. *S. molle* is distributed, in Mexico, by the states of Aguascalientes, Chiapas, Coahuila, Federal District, Durango, Guanajuato, Guerrero, Hidalgo, State of Mexico, Jalisco, Michoacán, Morelos, Nuevo León, Oaxaca, Puebla, Querétaro, San Luis Potosí, Sinaloa, Tlaxcala, Veracruz, and Zacatecas. It is also naturalized in California, the Canary Islands, and China [61, 62]. It has been reported that the leaves of the *Schinus molle* plant serve to remedy respiratory diseases and for the treatment of skin wounds. For its part, the resin is also used to treat oral conditions [51, 60]. No works have been found on the compounds present in the leaves of the *Schinus molle* plant to which an antibacterial action against *S. aureus* can be attributed in an alcoholic extract.

4.5 Inhibition of *Staphylococcus aureus* with extracts of anacahuita (*Cordia boissieri*), governor (*Larrea tridentata*), ash (*Leucophyllum frutescens*), and pirul (*Schinus molle*) with potential application in active packaging

4.5.1 Introduction

Staphylococcus aureus is recognized as one of the main pathogenic agents for humans [63]. This microorganism is a natural inhabitant of the man's skin without causing damage to it, but when the skin's defenses diminish, it can cause a disease [64]. *S. aureus* produces abscesses and superficial lesions of the skin and causes impetigo, septicemia, and fevers, besides producing infections in the nervous system, endocarditis, and osteomyelitis [63]. It also has an extraordinary ability to develop resistance to antimicrobials and has the potential to cause viable infections to be fatal. It is responsible for 32–47% of infections in the skin and subcutaneous tissue [65]. Annually *S. aureus* causes around 100,000 deaths in hospitalized patients in the USA [66]. Several research groups have focused their studies on the antimicrobial activity of various natural extracts. Medicinal plants are considered a potential source of new drugs because of their phytochemical content and their little toxic effect [67]. Molina-Salinas et al. reported that the methanolic extracts of *Cordia boissieri* and *Leucophyllum frutescens* show inhibitory activity against *Streptococcus pneumoniae* and *Mycobacterium tuberculosis*, respectively, and that the hexanic extract of *Schinus molle* exhibits inhibitory activity against *S. aureus* [68]. For its part, Tello-Baca reported that the aqueous extract of *Larrea tridentata* has inhibitory activity against *Escherichia coli* and *S. aureus* [69].

The objective of the present investigation was to evaluate if the alcoholic extracts of the plants of anacahuita (*Cordia boissieri*), governor (*Larrea tridentata*), ash

(*Leucophyllum frutescens*), and pirul (*Schinus molle*) exhibit antimicrobial activity against *S. aureus* and select those with potential use in the formulation of active food packaging.

4.5.2 Materials and methods

Vegetal material: The first variable of this research was the origin of the plant material. The plants were obtained in two ways: collection and purchase. The collection was carried out in the municipality of García, Nuevo León, and Mexico, and the purchase was made at the San Judas Hierbería in Monterrey, Nuevo León, Mexico.

Preparation of the extracts: The flowers of *C. boissieri* and the leaves of *L. frutescens*, *L. tridentata*, and *S. molle* were used to prepare the extracts. The plants were subjected to a fine grind in a porcelain mortar. The samples were passed through a sieve with 1 mm mesh. The second variable is the nature of the solvent (ethanol and methanol, at 70% v/v). The extracts were prepared at 6% (w/v). The extraction of the active compounds was carried out by soaking for 15 min at 35°C on a stirring and heating plate (PMC). The solutions were left to stand for 48 h at room temperature in hermetically sealed containers protected from light. The extracts were filtered on Panama flax cloth to remove large particles. Subsequently, the samples were centrifuged at 7000 rpm for 10 min. Finally, a filtration in a Kitasato flask with Whatman paper No. 4 was carried out. The obtained extracts were stored at 4°C in glass containers, hermetically sealed and covered against light.

Evaluation of inhibitory activity: The inhibitory activity was evaluated by the disk diffusion method in Trypticase Soy Agar (Becton Dickinson) (NCCLS, 2003). The tested extracts were purchased *C. boissieri* extracted with ethanol (ACE), purchased *C. boissieri* extracted with methanol (ACM), collected *C. boissieri* extracted with ethanol (ARE), collected *C. boissieri* extracted with methanol (ARM), purchased *L. frutescens* extracted with ethanol (CCE), purchased *L. frutescens* extracted with methanol (CCM), *L. frutescens* collected extracted with ethanol (CRE), *L. frutescens* collected extracted with methanol (CRM), purchased *L. tridentata* extracted with ethanol (GCE), purchased *L. tridentata* extracted with methanol (GCM), *L. tridentata* harvested extracted with ethanol (GRE), *L. tridentata* harvested extracted with methanol (GRM), purchased *S. molle* extracted with ethanol (PCE), purchased *S. molle* extracted with methanol (PCM), *S. molle* collected extracted with ethanol (PRE), and collected *S. molle* extracted with methanol (PRM). *S. aureus* (ATCC 6538) was used at a concentration of 10^8 CFU/ml. Plates were incubated at 37°C for 24 and 48 h. Negative controls were used for ethanol and methanol, as the extraction solvent, and as positive controls, kanamycin (50 mg/ml) and chloramphenicol (34 mg/ ml), because they are broad-spectrum antibiotics. The tests were done in triplicate. The statistical analysis, to select the best extract of each of the plants, was carried out using the Kruskal-Wallis test.

Minimum inhibitory concentration: The tube dilution method was used to determine the minimum inhibitory concentration of the selected extracts (NCCLS, 2000). Five concentrations of each extract (100, 200, 300, 400, and 500 μl) were placed in tubes with 5 ml of Trypticase Soy liquid medium (Becton Dickinson) with 500 μl of *S. aureus* (10^8 CFU/ml). The tubes were incubated at 37°C for 24 h. The tests were performed in triplicate. To determine if the inhibitory activity of the extracts is bactericidal or bacteriostatic, two tests were performed: (a) *S. aureus* (10^8 CFU/ml) in liquid medium of Trypticase Soybean (Becton Dickinson) was placed in 50/50 ratio with each one of the extracts was reseeded on Trypticase Soy Agar (Becton Dickinson) by the swab technique and incubated 24 h at 37°C and (b) a sample of bacterial cells from the inhibition halo formed was reseeded on Trypticase Soy Agar with striatum (Becton Dickinson) by each of the extracts and incubated at 37°C for 24 h. The tests were performed in triplicate. To select the two plants with the greatest inhibition, a statistical analysis was performed using the Kruskal-Wallis test.

Extract	Diameter of inhibition halo (mm)	
	24 h	**48 h**
ACE	8.33 ± 1.53	11.66 ± 2.89
ACM	10.00 ± 1.00	8.00 ± 1.00
ARE	11.00 ± 1.73	12.00 ± 2.00
ARM	11.67 ± 2.87	12.00 ± 1.00
CCE	7.33 ± 0.58	7.67 ± 1.15
CCM	9.33 ± 1.15	8.33 ± 2.31
CRE	10.67 ± 2.52	10.67 ± 1.52
CRM	8.00 ± 2.00	10.00 ± 2.00
GCE	10.00 ± 2.00	16.33 ± 1.15
GCM	14.33 ± 1.15	18.33 ± 2.89
GRE	17.00 ± 1.00	18.00 ± 1.00
GRM	11.33 ± 1.15	14.67 ± 0.58
PCE	10.00 ± 3.00	11.33 ± 3.79
PCM	15.67 ± 2.08	16.00 ± 1.73
PRE	16.67 ± 1.53	18.00 ± 2.65
PRM	16.67 ± 1.53	16.00 ± 3.00
Ethanol	6.50 ± 0.70	6.00 ± 0.50
Methanol	6.50 ± 0.70	6.00 ± 0.50
Kanamycin	7.30 ± 0.20	7.10 ± 0.10
Chloramphenicol	0	0

Table 2.
Diameters of the inhibition halo against S. aureus of the alcoholic extracts of C. boissieri, L. frutescens, L. tridentata, and S. molle plants.

Characterization of the extracts: The two selected extracts were analyzed by gas chromatography (Agilent 6890)/mass spectrometry (Agilent 5973) (GC/MS). An HP-5MS column (30 m × 0.25 mm × 0.25 mm) was used for the separation of the components. Helium as a carrier gas has a flow rate of 15 ml/min. The injection temperature was 270°C in "split" mode. The temperature of the column, after a period of 1 min at 80°C, was increased to 320°C at a rate of 15°C min^{-1}, and maintained at this temperature for 20 min. The mass spectrum had an ionization energy of 70 eV, a temperature of the ionization source of 230°C, and a quadrupole temperature of 150°C. The compounds were characterized with respect to the "Wiley7n.1" database.

4.5.3 Results

According to the obtained results in **Table 2**, we can observe that all alcoholic extracts of the plants *C. boissieri*, *L. frutescens*, *L. tridentata*, and *S. molle* have inhibitory activity against *S. aureus*. The tested extracts showed an increase in the diameter of the inhibition halo after 24–48 h (except for ACM and CCM extracts); this may be due to the fact that increasing the contact time increases the diffusion of the active compounds toward the middle. From the *C. boissieri* plant extracts, ACE (48 h), MCA (24 h), ARE (24 and 48 h), and MRA (24 and 48 h) showed a significantly higher inhibition than controls ($p < 0.05$), being the ARM extract (24 and 48 h) the one that showed the highest inhibitory activity against *S. aureus*.

Of the extracts of *L. frutescens*, CCM (48 h), CRE (24 and 48 h), and CRM (48 h) showed a significantly higher inhibitory activity than the controls ($p < 0.05$). CRE (24 and 48 h) was the extract with the highest inhibition against *S. aureus*. All evaluated extracts of *L. tridentata* showed a significantly higher inhibition than that of the controls ($p < 0.05$), presenting GRE (24 and 48 h) as the extract with greater inhibition against *S. aureus* and with a lower variance. In extracts of *S. molle*, PCM (24 and 48 h), PRE (24 and 48 h), and PRM (24 and 48 h) showed a significantly higher inhibition than that of the controls ($p < 0.05$), finding that PRE (24 and 48 h) is the extract with greater inhibitory activity against *S. aureus*.

Table 3 shows the minimum inhibitory concentration of the extract with the highest inhibition of each of the plants studied. The extract of the plant *L. tridentata* had the lowest minimum inhibitory concentration on *S. aureus* with 20 µl/ml, followed by the extract of *S. molle* with 80 µl/ml. Extracts of *C. boissieri* and *L. frutescens* had the highest minimum inhibitory concentration with 100 µl/ml each. It was also determined that the extracts of *L. tridentata* and *S. molle* have inhibitory activity against *S. aureus* of the bactericidal type and that the extracts of *C. boissieri* and *L. frutescens* show inhibitory activity of bacteriostatic type. **Figure 9** shows the comparison of the inhibition diameters of the extracts with greater inhibition of each of the plants studied. The GRE (24 and 48 h) and PRE (24 and 48 h) extracts have a significantly higher inhibitory activity than the ARM extracts (24 and 48 h) and CRE (24 and 48 h) ($p < 0.05$).

From GC/MS of *L. tridentata* extract (GRE), 12 compounds were identified, being 9,12-octadecanoic acid and 3,4′, 5,6,7-pentahydroxyflavone at 20.36 and 32.44 min, respectively, compounds they identified with greater certainty. Of the *S. molle* extract (PRE), 10 compounds were identified by GC/MS, with α-pinene compounds being

Extract	Minimum inhibitory concentration (µl/ml)
ARM	100
CRE	20
GRE	100
PRE	80

Table 3.
Minimum inhibitory concentration of the extracts of C. boissieri, L. frutescens, L. tridentata, and S. molle plants with the highest inhibition against S. aureus.

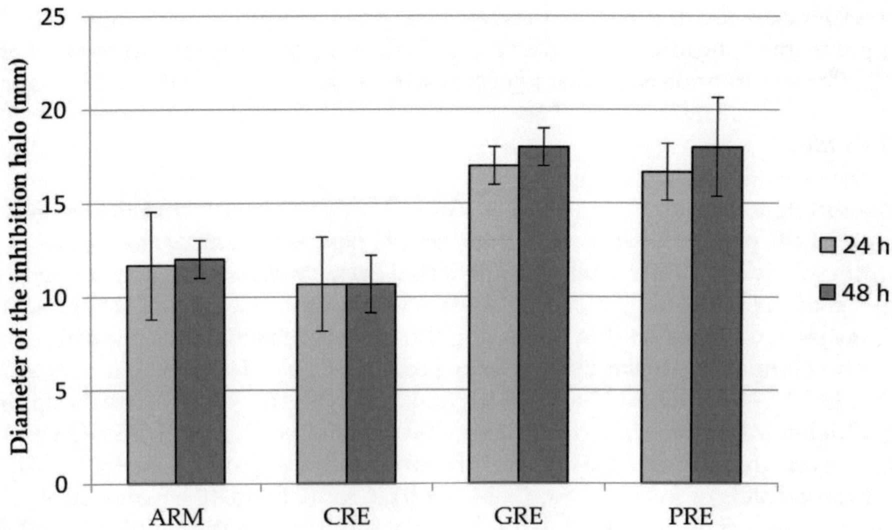

Figure 9.
Diameter of the inhibition halo of the extracts with greater inhibition against S. aureus of each of the plants C. boissieri, L. frutescens, L. tridentata, and S. molle. ARM, C. boissieri collected extracted with methanol; CRE, L. frutescens harvested extracted with ethanol; GRE, L. tridentata harvested extracted with ethanol; and PRE, S. molle harvested extracted with ethanol.

identified with greater certainty at 5.07 min, camphene at 5.30 min, p-mentha-1.5-comes at 6.12 min, p-mentha-1 (7), 2-diene at 6.51 min, 3 (15), 6-caryophylladiene at 12.15 min, 1 (10), 4 (15), 5-germacratriene a 12.92 min, 1 (10), 4-candinadiene at 13.39 min, 1.3-elemandien-11-ol at 13.71 min, and 4.9-cadinadiene at 16.27 min. The presence of 9, 12-octadecanoic acid and 3, 4 ', 5, 6, 7-pentahydroxyflavone was identified in the ethanolic extract of *L. tridentata* harvested and α-pinene; camphene; p-mentha-1, 5-diene; p-mentha-1 (7), 2-diene; 3 (15), 6-caryophyldiene; 1 (10), 4 (15), 5-germacratriene; 1 (10), 4-candinadiene; 1, 3-elemandien-11-ol; and 4, 9candinadiene in the ethanol extract of *S. molle* collected.

4.5.4 Discussion

For the four plants evaluated, there is greater inhibition in the extracts formulated with the harvested plants than with the purchased plants, since in the purchased plants, the storage time and the management that has been given are not known. In the extracts of the plants *L. frutescens*, *L. tridentata*, and *S. molle*, the ethanol was the solvent with which greater diameters were obtained in the inhibition zone. In the extracts of the *C. boissieri* plant, the solvent that allowed greater inhibition was methanol. The best inhibition results were obtained from the extracts of *L. tridentata* and *S. molle* plants. These plants represent a great antimicrobial potential; because as a plant that develops in arid conditions, it has a richness based on its biological specialization, since it is the product of thousands of years of physiological adaptation for its survival [50]. The inhibitory activity of *L. tridentata* can be attributed to the interaction of compounds present in the extracts, among which the 3,4′-5,6,7-pentahydroxyflavone exhibits an important role because the flavonoids are compounds with recognized antimicrobial activity [70]. The results obtained indicate that the four extracts exhibit antimicrobial activity, whether bactericidal or bacteriostatic. The activity observed was always greater than that of the controls (70% ethanol (E), kanamycin at a concentration of 50 mg/ml (K) and chloramphenicol at a concentration of 34 mg/ml (F)). Of the four extracts analyzed, that corresponding to *L. tridentata* showed the highest antimicrobial activity and the lowest minimum inhibitory concentration. The extract corresponding to *C. boissieri* showed the lowest antimicrobial activity and the highest minimum inhibitory concentration in relation to the other extracts.

The presence of 9, 12-octadecanoic acid and 3, 4 ', 5, 6, 7-pentahydroxyflavone was identified in the ethanolic extract of *L. tridentata* harvested and α-pinene; camphene; p-mentha-1, 5-diene; p-mentha-1 (7), 2-diene; 3 (15), 6-caryophyldiene; 1 (10), 4 (15), 5-germacratriene; 1 (10), 4-candinadiene; 1, 3-elemandien-11-ol; and 4, 9 candinadiene in the ethanol extract of *S. molle* collected.

In a previous work, Sáenz-Collins demonstrated that it was possible to obtain active antimicrobial PVOH biofilms against *S. aureus*, with potential use as dressings due to their biocompatibility. The extracts have no effect on the formation of biofilms. It was found that the higher the concentration of the extract in the biofilm, the greater the inhibition against *S. aureus*. Also, it was demonstrated that the alcoholic extracts had antimicrobial activity against Gram-negative bacteria as *Salmonella* and *E. coli* [71]. The drying temperature of the biofilm shows a diminishing effect on the antimicrobial activity; however, this remains present. It was demonstrated that the alcoholic extracts based on methanol and ethanol of *L. tridentata* show antimicrobial activity against *S. aureus* and that the ethanolic extract is more active. Sáenz-Collins also verified, through gas chromatography coupled to a mass spectrometer, that all the extracts of the governor plant possess an important amount of compounds with potential antimicrobial activity such as 4-vinylguaiacol, 4-hydroxybenzoic acid, and norisoguaiacin [71]. Although these plants can be purchased in some traditional local markets for medicinal use, their potential as a source of natural antimicrobial agents for use in active food packaging must be further investigated.

4.5.5 Conclusions

In the present work, it was demonstrated that the alcoholic extracts (ethanolic and methanolic) of the plants *C. boissieri*, *L. tridentata*, *L. frutescens*, and *S. molle* have inhibitory activity against *S. aureus*. The ethanolic extracts of the harvested plants show a greater halo of inhibition, being *L. tridentata* and *S. molle* the plants that present the best results. The results obtained indicate that the four extracts exhibit antimicrobial activity, whether bactericidal or bacteriostatic. Of the four extracts analyzed, that corresponding to *L. tridentata* showed the highest antimicrobial activity and the lowest minimum inhibitory concentration. The extract corresponding to *C. boissieri* showed the lowest antimicrobial activity and the highest minimum inhibitory concentration in relation to the other extracts. It was demonstrated that the antimicrobial activity of *L. tridentata* and *S. molle* is bactericidal and have potential use in active food packaging.

Author details

Cecilia Rojas de Gante*, Judith A. Rocha and Carlos P. Sáenz Collins
Departamento de Bioingeniería, Tecnológico de Monterrey, Campus Ciudad de México, Ciudad de México, Mexico

*Address all correspondence to: crd@itesm.mx

References

[1] Brody AL. Active packaging becomes more active. Food Technology. 2005;**12**:82-84

[2] Han JH. Antimicrobial food packaging. Food Technology. 2000;**54**(3):56-65

[3] Suppakul P, Miltz J, Sonneveld K, Bigger SW. Active packaging technologies with an emphasis on antimicrobial packaging and its applications. Journal of Food Science. 2003;**68**(2):408-420

[4] Vermeiren L, Devlieghere F, van Beest M, de Kruijf N, Debevere J. Developments in the active pakaging of foods. Trends in Food Science & Technology. 1999;**10**(3):77-86

[5] Lopez-Rubio A, Almenar E, Hernandez-Munoz P, Lagaron JM, Catala R, Gavara R. Overview of active polymer-based packaging technologies for food applications. Food Reviews International. 2004;**20**(4):357-387

[6] Alvarez García LY. Películas flexibles a base de sorgo (*Sorghum bicolor* Moench) como alternativa a envases plásticos y evaluación de sus propiedades barrera y mecánica [ITESM Tesis de Maestría]. Monterrey, N.L.: Centro de Biotecnología ITESM; 1999

[7] Schause AP. Envases biopoliméricos activos en nisina obtenidos a partir de almidón y harina de sorgo (*Sorghum bicolor* Moench) [Tesis de Maestría]. Monterrey N.L., México: Centro de Biotecnología ITESM; 2002

[8] Schause A, Rojas de Gante C. Active edible films from sorghum starch and flour with nisin. In: Worldpak 2002. Improving the Quality of Life through Packaging Innovation. Proceedings of the 13th IAPRI Conference on Packaging. Vol. I, Book 2. East Lansing (USA); 2002. pp. 819-825

[9] Valderrama-Solano AC, Rojas de Gante C. Two different processes to obtain antimicrobial packaging containing natural oils. Food and Bioprocess Technology. 2012;**5**:2522-2528

[10] Wang Y, Padua GW. Tensile properties of extruded zeinsheets and extrusion blown films. Macromolecular Materials and Engineering. 2003;**288**(11):886-893

[11] Corradini E, Felix AJ, Da Silva AA, Marcondes JA, Caparelli LH. Preparation and characterization of thermoplastic starch/zein blends. Materials Research. 2007;**10**(3):227-231

[12] Di Maio E, Mali R, Iannace S. Investigation of thermoplasticity of zein and kafirin proteins: Mixing process and mechanical properties. Journal of Polymers and the Environment. 2010;**18**(4):626-633

[13] Espino-Díaz M, Ornelas-Paz J, Martinez-Tellez MA, Santillán C, Barbosa-Cánovas GV, ZamudioFlores PB, et al. Development and characterization of edible films based on mucilage of *Opuntiaficus-indica* (L.). Journal of Food Science. 2010;**75**(6):E347-E352

[14] Bower CK, McGuire J, Daeschel MA. Influences of the antimicrobial activity of surface adsorbed nisin. Journal of Industrial Microbiology. 1995;**15**:227-233

[15] Ríos-Licea J. Envases biopoliméricos activos en sorbato de potasio y extractos naturales de orégano y ajo obtenidos a partir de harina de sorgo (*Sorghum bicolor* Moench) y evaluación de su actividad antimicrobiana frente a S.typhimurium, L.monocytogenes y *E. coli* [Tesis de Maestría]. Monterrey N.L., México: Centro de Biotecnología ITESM; 2008

[16] Tinoco-Pérez B. Cuantificación de antocianinas en envases biopolimericos activos con potencial acción antioxidante a partir de harina de maíz azul (*Zea mais* amilacea) [Tesis de Maestría]. Monterrey, N.L.: Tecnológico de Monterrey; 2007

[17] SAGARPA. Producción de Maíz en México [Internet]. 2009. Available from: http://www.sagarpa.gob.mx/agricultura

[18] SIAP. Cierre de la producción agrícola por cultivo [Internet]. 2009. Available from: http://www.siap.gob.mx/index.php?option=com_wrapper&view=wrapper&Itemid=350

[19] De la Rosa-Millán J. Análisis fisicoquímico, estructural y molecular de almidones de diferentes variedades de maíz azul [Tesis Maestría en Ciencias en desarrollo de productos bióticos]. Yautepec (México): Instituto Politécnico Nacional, Dependencia; 2009. pp. 1-12

[20] Dawson PL, Hirt DE, Rieck JR, Acton JC, Sotthibandhu A. Nisin release from films is affected by both protein type and film-forming method. Food Research International. 2003;**36**(9-10):959-968

[21] Pushpadass HA, Marx DB, Hanna AM. Effects of extrusion temperature and plasticizers on the physical and functional properties of starch films. Starch-Starke. 2008;**60**(10):527-538

[22] Wang Y, Rakotonirainy AM, Padua GW. Thermal behavior of zein-based biodegradable films. Starch-Starke. 2003;**55**(1):25-29

[23] López OV, Zaritzky NE, García MA. Physicochemical characterization of chemically modified corn starches related to rheological behavior, retrogradation and film forming capacity. Journal of Food Engineering. 2010;**100**(1):160-168

[24] Zeng M, Huang Y, Lu L, Fan L, Lourdin D. Effects of filler-matrix morphology on mechanical properties of corn starch-zein thermomoulded films. Carbohydrate Polymers. 2011;**84**(1):323-328

[25] Yang Q, Lue A, Qi H, Sun Y, Zhang X, Zhang L. Properties and bioapplications of blended cellulose and corn protein films. Macromolecular Bioscience. 2009;**9**(9):849-856

[26] Financiera Rural. Monografía del Sorgo [Internet]. Available from: http://www.financierarural.gob.mx/informacionsectorrural/Documents/Monografias/MonografiaSorgo%28jun11%29.pdf

[27] U.S. Grains Council. Sorghum [Internet]. 2010. Available from: http://www.grains.org/index. php?option=com_content&view=article&id=74&Itemid=120

[28] Rojas de Gante C, Rios-Licea J, Tinoco-Pérez B. Method for producing biofilms from cereal grains, biofilms obtained said method and use thereof for producing receptacles for containing and preserving foods. Patent No. WO2010/024657 A1. 2010

[29] Parra D, Tadini C, Ponce P, Lugao A. Mechanical properties and water vapor transmission in some blends of cassava starch edible films. Carbohydrate Polymers. 2004;**58**(4):475478

[30] Cecilia Rojas-de G, Grissel Trujillo-de S, Carlos Patricio Sáenz C, Andrea Valderrama S. Desempeño de una película de maíz azul en el envasado de un queso de humedad intermedia. Revista de Biotecnologia en el Sector Agropecuario y Agroindustrial Ed. Especial No. 2. 2013:49-58

[31] Valderrama Solano AC, Rojas de Gante C. Development of biodegradable films based on blue corn flour with potential applications in food packaging.

Effects of plasticizers on mechanical, thermal, and microstructural properties of flour films. Journal of Cereal Science. 2014;**60**:60-66

[32] Trujillo-de Santiago G, Rojas-de Gante C, García-Lara S, Verdolotti L, Di Maio E, Iannace S. Strategies to produce thermoplastic starch–zein blends: Effect on phase compatibilization. Journal of Polymers and the Environment. 2015;**22**(4):508-524

[33] Trujillo-de Santiago G, Rojas-de Gante C, García-Lara S, Verdolotti L, Di Maio E, Iannace S. Thermoplastic processing of blue maize and white sorghum flours to produce Bioplastics. Journal of Polymers and the Environment. 2015;**23**(1):72-82

[34] Valderrama ACS, Rojas de GC. Traceability of active compounds of essential oils in antimicrobial food packaging using a chemometric method by ATR-FTIR. American Journal of Analytical Chemistry. 2017;(8):726-741

[35] MacDonald PDM, Whitwam RE, Boggs JD, MacCormack JN, Anderson KL, Reardon JW, et al. Outbreak of listeriosis among Mexican immigrants as a result of consumption of illicitly produces Mexican-style cheese. Clinical Infectious Diseases. 2005;**40**:677-682

[36] Indu MN, Hatha AAM, Abirosh C, Harsha U, Vivekanandan G. Antimicrobial activity of some of the South-Indian spices against serotypes of *Escherichia coli*, *Salmonella*, *Listeria monocytogenes* and *Aeromonas hydrophila*. Brazilian Journal of Microbiology. 2006;**37**:153-158

[37] Martínez LM, Videa M, Mederos F, Mesquita J. Constructing a high-sensitivity, computerinterfaced, differential thermal analysis device for teaching and research. Journal of Chemical Education. 2007;**84**(7):1222-1223

[38] Rojas JJ, García AM, López AJ. Evaluación de dos metodologías para determinar la actividad antimicrobiana de plantas medicinales. BLACMA. 2005;**4**(2):28

[39] Pasterán F, Galas M. Manual de procedimientos, Sensibilidad a los antimicrobianos en Salmonella, Shigella y *E. coli*. Centro Regional de Referencia WHO- Global Salm. Surv. Para América del Sur. 2008

[40] Suppakul P, Sonneveld K, Bigger SW, Miltz J. Efficacy of polyethylene-based antimicrobial films containing principal consituents of basil. LWT Food Science and Technology. 2008;**41**:779-788

[41] Norma Oficial Mexicana NOM-110-SSA1-1994 – Bienes y servicios. Preparación y dilución demuestras de alimentos para su análisis microbiológico

[42] Ponce-Cevallos P, Buera M, Elizalde B. Encapsulation of cinnamon and thyme essential oils components (cinnamaldehyde and thymol) in β-cyclodextrin: Effect of interactions with water on complex stability. Journal of Food Engineering. 2010;**99**(1):70-75

[43] Dahmane M, Athman F, Sebih S, Guermouche MH, Bayle JP, Boudah S. Effect of the chain length on the thermal and analytical properties of laterally biforked nematogens. Journal of Chromatography A. 2010;**1217**(42):6562-6568

[44] Holland BJ, Hay JN. The thermal degradation of poly (vinyl alcohol). Polymer. 2001;**42**:67756783

[45] Rocha J. Desarrollo de películas de alcohol polivinílico (PVOH) con aceites esenciales naturales, para ser usados como "pads" (almohadillas) activos antimicrobianos en el envasado de quesos de cabra [Tesis de Maestría]. Monterrey N.L., México: Centro de Biotecnología ITESM; 2011

[46] Ultee A, Bennik MHJ, Moezelaar R. The phenolic hydroxyl group of carvacrol is essential for action against the food-borne pathogen *Bacillus cereus*. Applied and Environmental Microbiology. 2002;**68**(4):1561-1568

[47] Burt S. Essential oils: Their antibacterial properties and potential applications in foods, a review. International Journal of Food Microbiology. 2004;**94**:223-253

[48] Lambert RJW, Skandamis PN, Coote PJ, Nychas GJE. Study of the minimum inhibitory concentration and mode of action of oregano essential oil, thymol and carvacrol. Journal of Applied Microbiology. 2001;**91**:453-462

[49] Vázquez-Yanes C, Batis-Muñoz AI, Alcocer-Silva MI, Gual-Díaz M, Sánchez-Dirzo C. Árboles y arbustos potencialmente valiosos para la restauración ecológica y la reforestación. Reporte técnico del proyecto J084. CONABIO - Instituto de Ecología, UNAM; 1999

[50] Lira-Saldivar RH. Estado actual del conocimiento sobre las propiedades biocidas de la Gobernadora [*Larrea tridentata* (D.C.) Coville]. Revista Mexicana de Fitopatología. 2003;**21**(2):214-222

[51] Adame J, Adame H. Plantas curativas del noreste mexicano. Monterrey: Ediciones Castillo; 2000

[52] García-Llamas F. La gran enciclopedia de las plantas curativas. México: Editorial Diana; 2005

[53] Bronfman M. Nuevos Factores de Transcripción Nuclear. Santiago: Pontificia Universidad Católica de Chile; 2002

[54] Bruneton J. Farmacognosia: fitoquímica, plantas medicinales. Zaragoza: Acribia; 2001

[55] FDA/CFSAN. Illnesses and Injuries Associated With the Use of Selected Dietary Supplements. Miami: Dockets Management Branch Food and Drug Administration; 1993

[56] Alvarado MA, Foroughbakhch R, Jurado E, Rocha A. Caracterización morfológica y nutricional del fruto de anacahuita (*Cordia boissieri*) en dos localidades del Noreste de México. Phyton, International Journal of Experimental Botany. 2004;**73**:85-90

[57] Hernández-Magaña R, Gally-Jorda M. Plantas medicinales. México: Árbol Editorial; 1981

[58] Irish M. Trees and Shrubs for the Southwest. China: Congrees; 2008

[59] Villegas-Durán G, Bolaños-Medina A, Miranda-Sánchez JA, García-Aldape J, Galván-García OM. Flora nectarífera y polinífera en el estado de Tamaulipas. México: SAGARPA; 2003

[60] Hernández-Vázquez J, Sánchez-González S, González-Pacheco C, Luna-Peñaloza SR, Durán-Carmona V, Toledo-Ocampo A, Rodríguez-Velasco A, González-Lorenzo JR. Programa ambiental de la Universidad Autónoma de la Ciudad de México. 2011. Recuperado de: http://desarrollo.uacm.edu.mx.html

[61] Rzedowski GC, Calderón J. Flora del Bajío y regiones adyacentes. Pátzcuaro: Instituto de Ecología-Centro regional del Bajío; 1999

[62] Villaseñor JL, Espinosa FJ. Catálogo de malezas de México. México: UNAM; 1998

[63] Ruocco E, Donnarumma G, Baroni A, Tufano MA. Bacterial and viral skin diseases. Dermatologic Clinics. 2007;**25**(4):663-676

[64] Richardson AR, Libby SJ, Fang FC. A nitric oxide-inducible lactate dehydrogenase enables *Staphylococcus aureus* to resist innate immunity. Science. 2008;**319**(5870):1672-1676

[65] Diekema DJ, Pfaller MA, Schmitz FJ, Smayevsky J, Bell J, Jones RN. Survey of infections due to Staphylococcus species: Frequency of occurrence and antimicrobial susceptibility of isolates collected in the United States, Canada, Latin America, Europe, and the Western Pacific region for the SENTRY antimicrobial surveillance program, 1999. Clinical Infectious Diseases. 2001;**32**(2):S114-S132

[66] Demain A, Sánchez S. Microbial drug discovery: 80 years of progress. The Journal of Antibiotics. 2009;**62**:5-16

[67] Beg AZ, Ahmad I. Effect of *Plumbago zeylanica* extract and certain curing agents on multidrug resistant bacteria of clinical origin. World Journal of Microbiology and Biotechnology. 2000;**16**(8-9):841-844

[68] Molina-Salinas GM, Pérez-López A, Becerril-Montes P, Salazar-Aranda R, Said-Fernández S, Waksman-de Torres N. Evaluation of the flora of Northern Mexico for in vitro antimicrobial and antituberculosis activity. Journal of Ethnopharmacology. 2007;**109**(3):435-441

[69] Tello-Baca R. Actividad antibacteriana de plants con actividad hemaglutinante [QFB dissertation]. Morelia, México: Universidad Michoacana de San Nicolás de Hidalgo; 2009

[70] Cushnie T, Lamb AJ. Antimicrobial activity of flavonoids. International Journal of Antimicrobial Agents. 2005;**26**:343-356

[71] Sáenz-Collins CP. Aprovechamiento de la planta gobernadora (*Larrea tridentata*) para la obtención de un agente activo antimicrobiano frente a *Staphylococcus aureus* con aplicación en biopelículas de alcohol polivinílico para uso médico en forma de apósitos [Tesis] (Maestría en Ciencias). 2009

Chapter 4

Protein-Based Active Film as Antimicrobial Food Packaging: A Review

Nurul Saadah Said and Norizah Mhd Sarbon

Abstract

This review discusses the protein-based active film as antimicrobial food packaging derived from various sources such as gelatin, casein, whey and zein-based protein. The films properties that exhibit antimicrobial activity are being reviewed along with their application in food packaging industry. This paper also studies the inhibition activity by antimicrobial agents from organic and metallic sources which were incorporated into the protein-based film. Nowadays, protein-based film has emerged as one of the most extensively studied in food packaging sector as it exhibits good mechanical, optical, and oxygen barrier properties. In addition, protein-based film also showed good compatibility to polar surfaces while having effective control on the release of additives and bioactive compounds in food packaging system. This paper also detailed out information on antimicrobial food packaging in order to increase consumer awareness regarding food safety and healthy lifestyle while maintaining the quality and prolonged the shelf life of food product.

Keywords: protein, biopolymer, edible film, active packaging, antimicrobial agents

1. Food packaging

Food packaging is defined as a way of preparing food for transport, distribution, storage, and retailing till the end use while ensuring safe delivery to the ultimate customer [1]. Packaging systems are characterized into three groups which are primary, secondary, and tertiary packaging according to their layers or functions. Primary packaging is the first level of packaging which involves direct contact with the products. While secondary packaging contains a number of primary packages that protect the primary packages from damage during shipment and storage and are also designed to be displayed onto the retail shelves. As tertiary packaging, it acts as distribution carrier which consists of a number of secondary and primary packages [2]. Food packaging is designed to protect and maintain the quality and safety of foods from chemical, biological, and physical deterioration while helping in extending the product's shelf life [3]. In addition, its basic functions are commonly served as containment, protection or preservation, and communication and convenience purpose [1]. Packaging is also helpful in reducing municipal solid waste disposal and the cost of many food products by facilitating large-scale production and efficiency in bulk distribution. Food packaging also ensures the safety of products by decreasing the risk of tampering and adulteration [3].

IntechOpen

However, there are major drawbacks regarding non-biodegradable food packaging which caused environmental problems that include changes to the carbon dioxide cycle, composting problems, and increasing level of toxic emissions [4]. Stimulated by the environmental and growing interest of health safety concerns from consumers, many researchers have now been concentrating on ways to develop biodegradable packaging. Food packaging from biodegradable polymers have raised attention due to their renewable and environmental-friendly characteristics. Studies from renewable of natural biopolymers sources were included from polysaccharides (starch and chitin), lipids (waxes and paraffin), proteins (collagen and gelatin), or the combination of these components [5–7]. Among those, protein possessed greater characteristics and potential in food packaging due to its ability in film-forming process with high mechanical and barrier properties [8].

2. Protein-based food packaging

Proteins are composed of amino acid chains linked by peptide bonds to form a primary structure [9]. It can be characterized according to its amino acid composition, geometrical conformation, solubility, molecular weight, sedimentation behavior, surface polarity, and native molecular configuration shape [10]. Protein generally existed in two main classes that are known as fibrous or globular proteins. Fibrous and globular proteins have different sizes, shapes, solubility, appearances, and functions. Fibrous protein served as the main structural materials of animal tissues, while the globular proteins have multiple functions such as formation of enzymes, cellular messengers, and amino acids. Fibrous proteins consist of repetition of a single unit to form chains that act as connective tissues and associated closely with each other in parallel structures to provide strength and joint mobility, while globular proteins consist of long chains with numerous branches and folded into complicated spherical structures held together by a combination of hydrogen, ionic, hydrophobic, and covalent (disulfide) bonds. The example of fibrous protein that has gained great attention in studies of food packaging material is collagen. As for the globular protein, many research have been conducted on the use of casein, wheat gluten, corn zein, soy protein, whey protein, and mung bean protein as a great potential to be utilized as edible food packaging [11]. In food packaging, protein is mainly used as it exhibits good mechanical, optical, and oxygen barrier properties. Furthermore, protein is able to promote good compatibility to polar surfaces and control the release of additives and bioactive compounds in food packaging system [8, 10]. Therefore, many research have been keen to produce protein-based packaging that emerge in the form of edible films and coatings from various protein sources such as gelatin, casein, whey, corn zein, pea, wheat gluten, amaranth, soy, mung bean, and peanut.

2.1 Protein-based edible film

Nowadays, biodegradable film for food packaging has drawn attention from many researchers as an alternative approach to solve the problem arise from petroleum-based polymeric material that possesses non-biodegradability properties which leads to a critical environmental issue and causes exhaustion of natural resources. Natural biopolymers such as protein are eco-friendly and exhibit nontoxic properties which also have comparable physicochemical characteristics with the synthetic polymeric film [12]. In general, edible film is defined as a standalone thin layer sheet formed from a biopolymer matrix and possessed structural integrity. It served as a moisture barrier or as a solute/gas barrier while being able to improve the mechanical and rheological characteristics of the intended products [13]. These films also help in improving product quality by imparting certain functions such as antioxidant, antimicrobials, or any other specific functions while providing physical protection and extending the shelf life of the food products.

Protein-based films have been extensively utilized due to their relative abundance and good film-forming ability, contain high nutritional value, as well as provide desirable mechanical, gas barrier, and transparency properties [14]. Other than that, protein-based films also showed better mechanical properties than polysaccharide- and lipid-based films due to their unique structure that provides wider range of functional properties especially exhibiting a high intermolecular binding potential that is able to form a bond at a different position [14]. As widely known, protein-based edible film is being utilized from various kinds of protein sources which are mainly classified into two categories: animal and agro-based protein polymers. Several studies that have been conducted on animal-derived protein polymer include collagen, gelatin, fish myofibrillar protein, and whey protein, while the studies on agro-based protein polymer include the sources derived from corn zein, pea, wheat gluten, amaranth, soy, mung bean, and peanut.

The most preferred method to form edible protein-based film is by using solvent casting. The films are formed from solutions or dispersions of the protein as the solvent/carrier evaporates. The solvent/carrier is generally limited to water, ethanol, or ethanol-water mixtures [11]. The method was technically done by spreading dilute film solution and plasticizer into Petri dish or plates and drying them under ambient conditions or controlled relative humidity. Commonly, large-scale production uses more sophisticated equipment that is able to generate larger protein films by mechanically spreading the solution to a fixed thickness. There are several parameters that need to be determined for continuous film production such as air temperature, surface properties of the substrate upon which the films are formed, flow rate, and drying time. The films can be dried under ambient conditions by using several methods that are hot air, infrared energy, or microwave energy. The physical properties of the final film regarding film morphology, appearance, and barrier and mechanical properties can be significantly affected by the drying method used [15]. The other alternative method for protein-based film forming is by using extrusion. Extrusion process used elevated temperature and shear in order to soften and melt the polymer and thus allow the cohesive film matrix to form. The use of extrusion has certain advantages over solvent casting method as it is able to reduce more time and energy inputs as well as raise the cost of biopolymer film formation into a competitive range that is able to match and compete with the synthetic film production [15].

2.2 Protein-based edible coating

Meanwhile, edible coating is a more thinly edible film which is being formed directly onto the food or materials surface [16]. Edible coating can improve the physical and chemical integrity of the product by creating a modified overhead atmosphere and prevent the migration of moisture, oxygen, carbon dioxide, or any other solutes. It also acts as a carrier in terms of food additives (antioxidants, antimicrobials, and specific nutrients) while increasing the shelf life of the product. Furthermore, edible coatings can improve the product's appearance by adding color or gloss which seem to be more appealing to consumers [13, 16].

Protein coating is often being processed by using two common methods that are known as wet and dry (mainly extrusion) processes that depend on the target structure either mono- or multilayer structure. Wet coatings from polymer solutions or suspensions are commonly done by using lacquering or spraying techniques. Rheological properties of the coating formulation are greatly influenced by the techniques that will be used for wet coating process. Different types of methods are applicable for the drying process such as drying under ambient conditions, hot air, infrared energy, or microwave energy. The protein coating properties that include morphology, appearance, and barrier and mechanical properties will be influenced by the drying method used. As for dry process, extrusion method is one of the most common techniques that is being applied in conventional industrial method for protein coating. An extruder works by allowing the polymer to melt at high temperature during a relatively short time. The mechanical action of the screw and temperature exerts the material to melt, convey, compress, shear, mix, undergo variation of its amorphous content, optionally react, and be finally shaped through a die of a desired shape [10].

The protein-based film and coating were commonly being tested on their mechanical (tensile strength, elongation at break, and Young's modulus), barrier, (water vapor permeability and oxygen permeability), and physical (color and transparency) properties. However, due to its hydrophilic nature, protein-based film and coating also have high sensitivity to moisture and poor water vapor barrier properties. Thus, many studies have been conducted in order to improve and modify the functionality of protein-based film and coating as food packaging which includes the addition of different substances or agents such as cross linkers, plasticizers, and additives with antioxidant and antimicrobial properties. The incorporation of certain additives into packaging systems that intended to maintain or extend the quality of product or shelf life is referred as active packaging [17].

3. Active packaging

Active packaging is a medium which allows the interaction between the packaging, product, and environment. These systems involved the chemical, physical, and biological activities which change conditions of the packed food and help in extending the product's sustainability and shelf life. Moreover, active packaging is also able to enhance the microbiological safety and the sensory properties while maintaining the quality of the intended product [18]. Commonly, active packaging systems are concerned with substances that absorb (scavengers) or release (emitters) gases or steam which actively modifies the atmosphere inside packaging. Scavengers are used to remove unwanted items that commonly involved with the absorption of oxygen, ethylene, moisture, carbon dioxide, and flavors/odors from the environment into the internal packaging, while emitters are designed to release desired items that have a positive impact on food into the packaging environment that are commonly associated with the emitter of carbon dioxide, antimicrobial agents, antioxidants, and flavors [18]. Among those, antimicrobial packaging has been considered as the most promising method which incorporated antimicrobial agents into food packaging system that help in controlling the undesirable growth of a microorganism while extending the product's safety and shelf life [19]. As protein structure is comprised of hydrophilic nature, it can allow the control release of additive and bioactive compounds which make the protein-based film as one of the most promising media to be used in designated active antimicrobial packaging application.

3.1 Protein-based film as active packaging

Protein-based edible films were usually made from protein solutions or dispersions as the solvent/carrier evaporates. The solvent/carrier is normally composed of either water, ethanol, or ethanol-water mixtures [11]. Even though they exhibit poor water resistance, however, they are better when compared to polysaccharides in film-forming ability with good mechanical and barrier properties [20]. Protein-based film as active antimicrobial packaging is designed based on the diffusion of incorporated antimicrobial compounds to the product's surface while aiming to extend the shelf life period [21]. The antimicrobial activity depends on the rate of active compound diffusion by the antimicrobial agents which depends on several factors such as chemical compatibility with polymer matrix, headspace humidity, the physicochemical properties of the product which is being tested on, antimicrobial solubility in tested food, and also the released temperature [21]. Active antimicrobial packaging from protein-based edible films can be derived from various sources such as gelatin, casein, whey, corn zein, and wheat gluten.

3.1.1 Gelatin-based film as active packaging

Gelatin is a protein obtained by hydrolyzing the collagen contained in bones and skin of animals. Physical and chemical properties of the gelatin produced are greatly affected by the sources, age of animal, collagen type, and extraction method used [22]. The global gelatin production was 348.9 kilo tons in 2011 and is expected to reach 450.7 kilo tons in 2018, growing at a compound annual growth rate (CAGR) of 3.73% from 2012 to 2018 [23]. Among all protein sources, gelatin is being one of the most extensively studied due to its good filming properties while performing its duties to protect and extend the shelf life of food products. Many antimicrobial agents have been incorporated into a gelatin-based film such as metal ions, essential oils, natural extracts, polymers, organic acids, and bacteriocins which resulted in great inhibition toward growth of microorganism and pathogens.

For example, the gelatin-based active nanocomposite films containing silver nanoparticles (AgNPs) resulted in high antimicrobial activity against both Gram-negative (*Escherichia coli*) and Gram-positive (*Listeria monocytogenes*) bacteria. The bacterial inhibition might be due to the interaction of AgNPs with phosphorous and sulfur binding to microbial DNA and prevents bacterial replication which leads to cell death [24]. While, gelatin-based film with incorporation of oregano essential oil is found to be effective against Gram-negative (*Salmonella enteritidis* and *Escherichia coli*) and Gram-positive (*Staphylococcus aureus* and *Listeria monocytogenes*) bacteria. These antimicrobial properties might be attributed by the presence of two phenols (carvacrol and thymol) and monoterpene hydrocarbons (p-cymene and γ-terpinene) compounds which are present in oregano essential oils [25]. Based on another study, the incorporation of citric acid into the gelatin-based film also showed reduction of growth for Gram-negative bacteria (*Escherichia coli*) [26]. Citric acid has pKa 4.8 that makes cell membrane become permeable and allows the acid to enter the cell. Upon entering the cytoplasm, the acid will dissociate, thus lowering the internal pH of the cell which leads to disruption of cellular functions of a microorganism [27]. Based on the results of this study, it showed that gelatin with the incorporation of antimicrobial agents has resulted in excellent properties as active antimicrobial food packaging as they managed to inhibit microbial growth of the food product. Thus, it can be concluded that gelatin-based film has emerged as one of the most widely studied biopolymer in film processing sector as compared to other sources of protein-based film while showing great potential as a medium to release or emit active antimicrobial agents against growth of microorganism and pathogens.

3.1.2 Casein-based film as active packaging

Casein-based edible film production also has been numerously studied because they displayed high nutritional quality with good sensory properties. Casein is commonly found in mammalian milk or in dairy products. Casein proteins comprise 80% of the total protein content in milk which precipitated from skim milk by acidifying the milk to produce acid casein to its isoelectric point of approximately 4.6 or the milk is treated with rennet to produce rennet casein. The casein is then being separated, washed, and dried [11, 28]. Casein is mainly comprised of three principal components, α, β, and κ, that formed colloidal micelles in milk which contains numerous amounts of casein molecules that are being stabilized by a calcium-phosphate bridge [11]. Due to excellent functional properties and natural abundant sources, caseins are used in numerous manufactured products such as in bakery applications, beverages, milk product, snack foods, edible films, etc. Casein or caseinates in the world market used in the food industry were reported in the range between 200,000 and 2,500,000 tons [28]. Caseins and caseinates can be prompted into edible films from aqueous solutions. Edible casein films are able to form a good barrier against oxygen and other nonpolar molecules because casein helps in supplying a great quantity of polar functional groups, such as hydroxyl and amino groups toward the film matrix. This property allows the casein film to be used as active packaging and can be combined with other packaging materials to protect products which are prone to oxidation or moisture [29].

In a study conducted by Arrieta et al. [30], sodium and calcium caseinate films with addition of carvacrol showed antibacterial effectiveness against both Gram-negative (*Escherichia coli*) and Gram-positive (*Staphylococcus aureus*) bacteria, while sodium caseinate-based edible film containing *Zataria multiflora Boiss*. essential oil exhibited a large inhibitory effect on Gram-positive (*Staphylococcus aureus*) followed by Gram-negative (*Salmonella Typhimurium* and *Escherichia coli*) bacteria [31]. Meanwhile, Oussalah et al. [32] mentioned that calcium caseinate and whey protein isolate edible films containing carboxymethyl cellulose with addition of 1% oregano essential oil showed inhibitory effect against Gram-negative bacteria that were *Escherichia coli* and *Pseudomonas* spp. on the surface of beefsteaks. The antimicrobial activity was mainly derived from phenolic compounds (carvacrol and thymol) which are present in the essential oil. The inhibition effect was done by interacting with the lipid bilayer of cytoplasmic membranes, causing them to be more permeable, which later induced and increased uptake of antibiotics by the bacterial cell [33]. From this study, it can be seen that caseinate film provides good matrices for the antimicrobial agent to release the active compounds that help to inhibit the growth of microorganisms.

3.1.3 Whey protein-based film as active packaging

Whey is a by-product derived from cheese-making process which is being defined as the remaining matter in the milk serum after coagulation of casein at pH 4.6 and temperature of 20°C. Whey protein is comprised of several individual proteins known as beta-lactoglobulin, alpha-lactalbumin, bovine serum albumin, and immunoglobulins [15]. The global whey protein market is projected to reach the compound annual growth rate (CAGR) of 7.5% from 2018 to 2023, and the demand was estimated at a value of $9.4 billion in 2017 [34]. The recovering process of whey solid component helps in reducing the organic pollution evolved from whey wastes while being able to optimally utilize the nutritional and functional properties provided by whey protein to be used in diverse sector [35]. The demand for whey protein among producers of food and beverages is increasing as they capitalize on the functional benefits of whey protein in various products such as sports nutrition, confectionery, bakery and ice cream products, infant formula, and health foods. Recent study has developed an alternative use of whey protein products to form edible film and coatings on surface of food products [36]. Whey protein-based films are found to exhibit clear, odorless with good barrier properties to oxygen and lipids [37]. They also provide good matrices which allow the combination with other packaging materials to enhance the film's functionality as an active film against microorganism or moisture.

A study reported that whey protein-based films incorporated with oregano and garlic essential oil resulted in larger inhibitory zones on Gram-negative (*Escherichia coli* and *Salmonella Enteritidis*) and Gram-positive bacteria (*Staphylococcus aureus*, *Lactobacillus plantarum*, and *Listeria monocytogenes*) [38], while another study of whey protein-based films incorporated with oregano essential oil showed antimicrobial activity against fungus species (*Penicillium commune*) [39]. The inhibition toward the microorganism was prompted by thymol and carvacrol compounds that are mainly present in essential oil. Based on another study of whey protein isolate (WPI) films supplemented with *Lactobacillus sakei*, the bacterial reductions were observed for Gram-negative (*Escherichia coli*) and Gram-positive bacteria (*Listeria monocytogenes*) after 36 hours and 120 hours of refrigerated storage on beef cube sample, respectively [40]. *Lactobacillus sakei* produced bacteriocin known as sakacin P which tends to exhibit antimicrobial properties [41]. Meanwhile, the incorporation of acetic, lactic, propionic, and benzoic acids (5%, v/v each) into whey protein-based edible film showed great inhibition zones against Gram-negative (*Escherichia coli* and *Salmonella* sp.) and Gram-positive bacteria (*Lactobacillus bulgaricus* and *Streptococcus thermophiles*) [42]. The use of acids causes acidification of growth media through acid dissociation into the cytoplasm which then induced the microbial inhibition [27]. Whey protein-based film also yields excellent results toward growth of microorganism as it provides good polymeric matrices for the antimicrobial agents to emit the active compounds into the packaging system.

3.1.4 Zein protein-based film as active packaging

Zein is a major protein in corn that is being classified as prolamin protein which dissolved in 70–80% ethanol. Zein is a relatively hydrophobic and thermoplastic material. The high content of nonpolar amino acids found in zein component might have an association with the hydrophobic nature of zein [11]. The corn is processed by using four different methods: wet-milling, dry milling, dry-grind processing, and alkaline treatment. After that, zein is being extracted from these products/coproducts of corn which could result in different properties and end uses. Corn wet-milling process yields a protein-rich coproduct called corn gluten meal (CGM) from which zein has been commercially extracted. The other methods are dry-milled corn (DMC) in which fibrous material is being separated from grits. As for the dry-grind ethanol process, the corn is ground along with the subsequent saccharification and fermentation of glucose to ethanol, leaving behind the coproduct distillers' dried grains with solubles (DDGS). Fractions such as cellulosic materials and protein are concentrated in DDGS due to conversion of starch to sugars and subsequently ethanol. While, alkaline treatment method has been mainly utilized for the use of human consumption and only has little basis for zein extraction. Most zein extractions have been based on aqueous alcohol extractions, but many other solvents were reported to be able to solubilize zein too [43]. A report by Informa Economics, Inc. [44] showed that zein was clarified as high-value product, and the cost for purified zein production had achieved $9–30/lb. Zein proteins have been found to serve good materials for coating in pharmaceutical products and food ingredients as they exhibit tough and hydrophobic grease-proof coating properties that make them resistant against microbial attacks. Other potential applications of zein include its usage in fiber, adhesive, coating, ceramic, ink, cosmetic, textile, chewing gum, and biodegradable plastics [45]. In addition, numerous studies have been conducted on utilization of zein protein on development of biodegradable films as it exhibits good film-forming properties. Zein film production involves the development of hydrophobic, hydrogen, and limited disulfide bonds between zein chains in the film matrix [11]. Moreover, zein also showed good properties as carrier for antimicrobial agents such as lysozyme, lactoperoxidase, glucose oxidase, bacteriocins, plant phenolics, and essential oils [20].

A study conducted by Moradi et al. [46] has proved that zein-based film showed excellent antimicrobial properties through the release time of antibacterial agent from the film matrix into minced meat. In this literature, the zein and *Zataria multiflora Boiss.* essential oil-incorporated film has resulted in effective inhibition against both Gram-negative (*Escherichia coli*) and Gram-positive bacteria (*Listeria monocytogenes*) during 3 days of storage at 4°C. The result obtained corresponded with the finding by Kashiri et al. [21] which stated that the results showed that films containing *Zataria multiflora Boiss*. essential oil at 5% (g of essential oil/g of dry zein powder) achieved reductions of 1.18 log and 1.14 log against Gram-positive (*Listeria monocytogenes*) and Gram-negative (*Escherichia coli*) bacteria, respectively. While, as the concentration *Zataria multiflora Boiss*. essential oil being increased to 10%, the log reduction value increased to 2.16 log and 2.65 log for films against Gram-positive (*Listeria monocytogenes*) and Gram-negative (*Escherichia coli*) bacteria, respectively. From this study, the antimicrobial effect can be explained by the major compound (thymol and carvacrol) found in *Zataria multiflora Boiss.* essential oil which prevents the further growth of microorganism. The study also focused on addition of monolaurin into zein-based film which resulted in effective antimicrobial activity against Gram-positive bacteria (*Listeria monocytogenes*) during 3 days of storage at 4°C. The inhibition effect toward microorganism by monolaurin is caused by the interference with cytoplasmic membrane of microorganisms [46]. In another study by Mei et al. [47], the antimicrobial activity of silver nanocluster (AgNCs) and $AgNO_3$- embedded zein film was tested on pathogenic *Escherichia coli*. The study showed that there were inhibition zones present with 1.95 and 2.05 mm at concentration of 10 μg Ag of AgNCs and $AgNO_3$, respectively. Silver particles exhibit great antimicrobial activity as they can bind to the bacterial cell wall and cell membrane and inhibit the respiration process of microorganisms, while for the case of *Escherichia coli* inhibition, silver inhibits the uptake of phosphate while releasing succinate, proline, phosphate, mannitol, and glutamine from *Escherichia coli* cells [48]. Thus, based on all the results obtained by this study, it can be concluded that zein-based film does result in good compatibility with incorporation of antimicrobial agents. This is because the antimicrobial agents are able to release the antimicrobial compound agent into the packaging system and managed to inhibit the growth of microorganism.

4. Antimicrobial agent in food packaging

Active antimicrobial packaging involved the continuous interaction with the food product over specific shelf life by actively altering the internal environment [49]. In antimicrobial packaging system, the prevention and reducing growth rate of microorganism by extending the lag period will occur once the antimicrobial agents have been acquired [50]. An extensive study discussed the incorporation of antimicrobial agents in food packaging system from various organic and inorganic sources such as natural extracts (green tea), essential oils (clove, oregano, and thyme), enzyme (lysozyme), polymer (chitosan), organic acid (acetic acid, lactic acid, and benzoic acid), bacteriocins (nisin), and metal ions (zinc oxide and silver nanoparticles). However, due to stability of organic sources when exposed to extreme temperature, their use and application as antimicrobial agents might be limited. Thus, inorganic metals have gained more interest as they are relatively more stable at higher temperatures [51].

4.1 Organic sources as antimicrobial agents

Organic sources of antimicrobial agents can be comprised of animal and plant origin, microbial metabolites, and organic acids. As majority of organic antimicrobials derived from natural origin, they are thus able to inactivate microorganisms and enzymes without affecting the organoleptic or nutritional properties of the food products.

4.1.1 Plant-derived antimicrobial agent

Plant-derived antimicrobial agents possessed phenolic compounds that are able to alter the permeability of microbial cell and interfere with cell membrane functionality such as electron transport, protein synthesis, nutrient uptake, and enzyme activity, while the phenolic compounds also allow the loss of biomolecules such as ribose and sodium glutamate from inside the cell [52]. A wide range of study on antimicrobial agents that derived from plant origin mainly discussed on essential oils and natural extracts. The antimicrobial activity of essential oils is based on their molecular hydrophobicity which allows strong interaction with the lipids of cell membrane through their existence of phenolic compounds. This action will then increase the permeability of cell membrane and disturb the functionality and structure of the cell which leads to leakage of ions and cytoplasmic content inside the cell [53].

In a study conducted by Yanwong and Threepopnatkul [54], the fish skin gelatin-edible films were incorporated with peppermint and citronella essential oils at different concentrations (10, 20, and 30%, w/w). The study showed that the incorporation of both essential oils exhibited excellent antibacterial properties against both Gram-negative (*Escherichia coli*) and Gram-positive (*Staphylococcus aureus*) bacteria. The inhibition activities were triggered by the presence of a major constituent in both essential oils that were identified as *p*-menthone and menthol and citronellal and citronellol for peppermint and citronella essential oils, respectively [55, 56]. While, Martucci et al. [57] observed the antimicrobial activity of oregano and lavender essential oils incorporated into gelatin film that were tested against *Escherichia coli* and *Staphylococcus aureus*. The study found that both essential oils exhibited good antimicrobial properties against the tested bacteria which were Gram-negative (*Escherichia coli*) and Gram-positive bacteria (*Staphylococcus aureus*) in concentrations above 2000 ppm. Oregano essential oil contained carvacrol and thymol, while lavender essential oil revealed a prevalence of linalool and camphor as their major compounds which exhibited good antimicrobial activity against tested microorganism. Another study mentioned that whey protein film with addition of 1–4% of cinnamon oil was tested against *Escherichia coli* and *Staphylococcus aureus*. However, the study showed antimicrobial activity only against *Staphylococcus aureus* with the highest inhibition zone at 4% addition of cinnamon oil into the whey protein film [58]. In addition, a major compound in cinnamon oil that exhibited the antimicrobial activity was identified as trans-cinnamaldehyde or cinnamaldehyde [59]. In the literature, it was mentioned that *Escherichia coli* exerted more resistance to cinnamon essential oil as compared to *Staphylococcus aureus*. This is due to the difference in bacteria's outer membrane structure. Gram-negative bacteria (*Escherichia coli*) possessed a thicker layer of the lipopolysaccharide outer membrane around the cell wall which is shown to be more resistant to hydrophobic substance of essential oil as compared with the Gram-positive (*Staphylococcus aureus*), which possesses single peptidoglycan layer structure [59]. Thus, from this study, it can be seen that all mentioned essential oils exhibited certain compounds that exerted good antimicrobial activity which could enhance the food product shelf life and stability.

4.1.2 Animal-derived antimicrobial agent

Antimicrobial agents originated from animal sources are commonly being used as they exhibited good resistance and inhibition toward growth of microorganism. They evolved as part of defense mechanisms in antimicrobial system. Most of the antimicrobial agents derived from animals emerged in the form of antimicrobial peptides such as pleurocidin, lactoferrin, defensins, and protamine [52]. These peptides were applicable as antibiotic resistant as they are able to destruct the cellular lipid bilayer membranes and can hinder even the fast-growing microorganism to mutate. Furthermore, they have good antimicrobial activity against both Gram-positive and Gram-negative bacteria while also showing antifungal and antiviral activities [60]. There are other effective antimicrobial enzymes which come from egg white, milk, and blood that are known as lysozyme. A study by Kaewprachu et al. [61] reported that minced pork wrapped with catechin-lysozyme which incorporated with gelatin film resulted in lower counts of total plate count, yeasts, and molds than minced pork that was wrapped with PVC film. The addition of lysozyme triggered the cleaving process of peptidoglycan in bacterial cell walls and resulted in lysis of bacterial cell. This result showed that catechin-lysozyme/gelatin film could inhibit the microbial growth, while there are also various studies on certain polysaccharides and lipids from animals that showed excellent antimicrobial activity. For example, Pisoschi et al. [52] stated that chitin derived from the exoskeletons of crustaceans, insects, mollusks, and the cell wall of microorganisms exhibited antimicrobial properties. Apart from that, chitosan which is obtained from the exoskeletons of crustaceans and arthropods and existed as a deacetylated form of chitin also showed effective antifungal and antibacterial activities [52]. In a literature studied by Malinowska-Pañczyk et al. [62], the incorporation of chitosan was observed on its ability as antimicrobial agent against Gram-negative (*Escherichia coli* and *Pseudomonas fluorescens*) and Gram-positive (*Staphylococcus aureus* and *Listeria innocua*) bacteria. The study then revealed all strains of bacteria were completely inactivated after 24 hours of incubation period for gelatin film incorporated with chitosan-90. As for gelatin films with addition of chitosan-73, the results showed that only *Pseudomonas fluorescens* and *Listeria innocua* were completely inactivated, while *Escherichia coli* and *Staphylococcus aureus* cells were partially inactivated after 24 hours of incubation. The inhibition factor was due to the cationic nature of chitosan which induced the electrostatic interaction between positively charged RN $(CH_3)_3^+$ sites and negatively charged microbial cell membranes which led to cellular lysis [63]. Therefore, it can be seen that antimicrobial agents derived from animals resulted good inhibitory effect against microorganism and can be applied in food packaging for enhancing shelf life and quality of intended products.

4.2 Metallic sources as antimicrobial agents

Metals have been widely used as antimicrobial agents for a long time due to their ability to cause injuries to microbial cells by exerting oxidative stress, protein dysfunction, or membrane damage [64]. Metal ions such as copper, silver, zinc, palladium, and titanium have been studied as active antimicrobial agents against a wide spectrum of bacteria, yeast, and fungi [65]. Due to stability of organic sources at higher temperature, their application in food packaging may be limited, thus giving great advantage to metallic sources that are more stable at higher temperature [51].

4.2.1 Zinc particles as antimicrobial agents

Zinc particle especially zinc oxide (ZnO) is being widely proposed to be used as antimicrobial agents with broad range of other applications due to their specialty to survive under harsh environment. The antimicrobial activity by zinc oxide (ZnO) particles were proposed due to emission of zinc ions (Zn^{2+}), which are able to penetrate into the bacteria's cell wall and affect the cytoplasmic content in the cell that leads to the death of bacteria. The incorporation of zinc oxide nanoparticles into gelatin was observed by Divya et al. [66] which revealed that the film showed higher inhibitory effect against Gram-negative bacteria (*Pseudomonas aeruginosa*) than Gram-positive (*Enterococcus faecalis*) bacteria. The results corresponded with the statement which suggested that ZnO induced photocatalytic mechanism related to the semiconductive properties of ZnO which lead to the formation of reactive oxygen species (ROS) and H_2O_2 which damaged the cell wall structure of bacteria [67, 68]. The literature by Pasquet et al. [67] also stated that the lipid bilayer membrane of Gram-negative bacteria was more sensitive toward reactive oxygen species (ROS) produced by ZnO particles than the thick membrane of Gram-positive bacteria that is coated by a peptidoglycan protective layer. Meanwhile, the study on gelatin/ZnO nanoparticles of nano-composite films showed great antibacterial activity against both Gram-positive (*Listeria monocytogenes*) and Gram-negative (*Escherichia coli*) foodborne pathogenic bacteria. The study discussed that the antimicrobial activity toward both Gram-negative and Gram-positive bacteria was due to the easy penetration of nanoparticles in the cytoplasmic content of the cell which then leads to death of cell [69]. Thus, it can be concluded that incorporation of zinc particles into protein-based film helps in exerting antimicrobial activity against foodborne pathogens.

4.2.2 Silver particles as antimicrobial agents

The application of silver particles has received great attention from the researchers from all over the world due to their wide spectrum and application in antimicrobial packaging. Silver is often used in the size of nanoparticles as they give more potent effect against foodborne pathogen due to their enhanced catalytic reactivity owing to its large surface area to volume ratio. Based on a study conducted by Kanmani and Rhim [24], the incorporation of silver nanoparticles (AgNPs) into gelatin film was tested against Gram-positive (*Listeria monocytogenes*) and Gram-negative (*Escherichia coli*) bacteria. The results mentioned that the AgNP/gelatin biocomposite film showed high-inhibitory effect against both tested microorganisms. This might be due the interaction of AgNPs with compounds of protein and DNA in the cell that contain phosphorous and sulfur which prevent DNA replication and cause death of the cell. Furthermore, some study suggested that positively charged AgNPs are able to bind with negatively charged bacterial cell membranes that cause disruption of cell walls by shrinkage of the cytoplasm and membrane detachment that led to cell death [70]. In this literature, it also stated that AgNPs could penetrate the bacteria which inactivate the enzymes and induce the production of H_2O_2 and cause cell to die [24]. Meanwhile, another study by Mei et al. [47] observed on the antimicrobial activity of silver nanocluster (AgNC)-embedded zein film against pathogenic *Escherichia coli*. The study showed that adding 10 μg of AgNCs into zein film resulted in great antimicrobial effect as indicated by inhibition zones of 1.95. In this literature, it stated that the inhibitory effect was influenced by the release rate of Ag that was embedded in zein films. Since AgNCs had high surface to volume ratio due to its ultra-small size, it thus led to greater surface contact with bacteria and consequently exhibited higher antimicrobial activity. Therefore, based on this study, it can be confirmed that addition of silver particles into protein-based film is able to exhibit mechanism of antibacterial action against microorganisms.

5. Application of protein-based active film in food packaging

Protein-based edible film has gained great interest due to its wide application as edible food packaging as compared to synthetic films. In addition, it is able to provide good matrix and acts as a medium for incorporation of antimicrobial and antioxidant agents into the film to release or emit their specific functions that help in enhancing the safety, stability, functionality, and shelf life of food products. Moreover, it also can be applied to control the diffusion rate of preservative substances from the product's surface to the internal environment of food. Meanwhile, protein-based packaging also is being extensively used as food wrapper and is being applied at the interfaces between different layers of heterogeneous food, while protein-based edible films could be used together with nonedible film as multilayer food packaging materials where it can be employed as internal layers that have direct contact with food materials [11]. Furthermore, due to good permeability against oxygen, carbon dioxide, and water vapor, protein-based film can be applied to the surfaces of fresh-cut food product in order to extend shelf life of the product by delaying color changes and ripening and prevent the effect of enzymatic browning and reducing moisture and aroma loss [71]. Thus, it can be concluded that protein-based edible film exhibits good characteristics through their mechanical and barrier properties as food packaging which is able to substitute the utilization synthetic film packaging.

6. Conclusion

Antimicrobial food packaging have gained great interest due to high inhibition of microbial activity that helps in prolonging the shelf life of packaged food and enhancing the food's safety while improving the functionality of the film. The incorporation of antimicrobial agents from various organic and inorganic sources into protein-based edible film has been discussed, and their effectiveness was mainly found depending on their activity against the target microorganism, the types of polymer used, the film's properties, and the factor based on the packaged food's composition, pH, water activity, as well as the storage and environmental condition. However, there are some challenges in creating good antimicrobial films that follow the regulatory and industry requirements which also aim in producing at low production cost and are able to meet with the consumer demands without altering the sensory characteristics of the intended packaged food. Therefore, more studies need to be done on biocomposite protein-based packaging films with incorporation of antimicrobial agents that might also require chemical, toxicological, and further test in securing more safe and approved products according to the standard food safety regulations while being able to deliver good means in protecting the safety and quality of packaged food.

Author details

Nurul Saadah Said and Norizah Mhd Sarbon*
School of Food Science and Technology, Universiti Malaysia Terengganu,
Kuala Nerus, Terengganu, Malaysia

*Address all correspondence to: norizah@umt.edu.my

References

[1] Shin J, Selke SEM. Food Packaging. Food Processing: Principles and Applications. 2nd ed. United States: John Wiley & Sons, Ltd; 2014

[2] Robertson GL. Packaging and Food and Beverage Shelf Life. Food and Beverage Stability and Shelf Life. Cambridge: Woodhead Publishing Limited; 2016

[3] Trinetta V. Definition and function of food packaging. In: Reference Module in Food Science. 2016:1-2

[4] Ezeoha SL, Ezenwanne JN. Production of biodegradable plastic packaging film from cassava starch. IOSR Journal of Engineering. 2013;**10**(5):14-20

[5] Hassan B, Chatha SAS, Hussain AI, Zia KM, Akhtar N. Recent advances on polysaccharides, lipids and protein based edible films and coatings: A review. International Journal of Biological Macromolecules. 2018;**109**:1095-1107

[6] Sarbon NM, Badii F, Howell NK. Preparation and characterisation of chicken skin gelatin as an alternative to mammalian gelatin. Food Hydrocolloids. 2013;**30**(1):143-151

[7] Vieira MGA, Silva MAD, Santos LOD, Beppu MM. Natural-based plasticizers and biopolymer films: A review. European Polymer Journal. 2011;**47**:254-263

[8] Zink J, Wyrobnik T, Prinz T, Schmid M. Physical, chemical and biochemical modifications of protein-based films and coatings: An extensive Review. International Journal of Molecular Sciences. 2016;**17**:1376

[9] Rostom H, Shine B. Basic metabolism: Proteins. Surgery. 2018;**36**(4):153-158

[10] Coltelli MB, Wild F, Bugnicourt E, Cinelli P, Lindner M, Schmid M, et al. State of the art in the development and properties of protein-based films and coatings and their applicability to cellulose based products: An extensive review. Coatings. 2016;**6**(1):1-59

[11] Wittaya T. Protein-based edible films: Characteristics and improvement of properties. In: Structure and Function of Food Engineering, InTech; 2012. pp. 43-71

[12] Gautam RK, Kakatkar AS, Karani MN. Development of protein-based biodegradable films from fish processing waste. International Journal of Current Microbiology and Applied Sciences. 2016;**5**(8):878-888

[13] Ramos OL, Fernandes JC, Silva SI, Pintado ME, Malcata FX. Edible films and coatings from whey proteins: A review on formulation, and on mechanical and bioactive properties. Critical Reviews in Food Science and Nutrition. 2012;**52**(6):533-552

[14] Kaewprachu P, Rawdkuen S. Mechanical and physico-chemical properties of biodegradable protein-based films: A comparative study. Food and Applied Bioscience Journal. 2014;**2**(1):14-29

[15] Dangaran K, Tomasula PM, Qi P. Structure and Function of Protein-Based Edible Films and coatings. Edible Films and Coatings for Food Applications. New York: Springer; 2009

[16] Jooyandeh H. Whey protein films and coatings: A review. Pakistan Journal of Nutrition. 2011;**10**(3):296-301

[17] Dobrucka R, Cierpiszewski R. Active and intelligent packaging food – research and development–A review. Polish Journal of Food and Nutrition Sciences. 2014;**64**(1):7-15

[18] Wyrwa J, Barska A. Innovations in the food packaging market: Active packaging. European Food Research and Technology. 2017;**243**:1681-1692

[19] Gonçalves AA, Rocha MDOC. Safety and quality of antimicrobial packaging applied to seafood. MOJ Food Processing and Technology. 2017;**4**(1):00079

[20] Mellinas C, Valdes A, Ramos M, Burgos N, Garrigos MDC, Jimenez A. Active edible films: Current state and future trends. Journal of Applied Polymer Science. 2016;**133**(2):42631

[21] Kashiri M, Cerisuelo JP, Domínguez I, Lopez-Carballo G, Muriel-Gallet V, Gavara R, et al. Zein films and coatings as carriers and release systems of *Zataria Multiflora* Boiss. Essential oil for antimicrobial food packaging. Food Hydrocolloids. 2017;**70**:260-268

[22] Gómez-Guillén MC, Giménez B, López-Caballero ME, Montero MP. Functional and bioactive properties of collagen and gelatin from alternative sources: A review. Food Hydrocolloids. 2011;**25**:1813-1827

[23] Transparency Market Research. Gelatin Market by Raw Material (Pig Skin, Bovine Hide, Bones and Others) for Food & Beverage, Nutraceuticals, Pharmaceuticals, Photography, Cosmetics and Other Applications–Global Industry Analysis, Size, Share, Growth, Trends and Forecast, 2012-2018;2013. Retrieved from: https://www.prnewswire.com/news-releases/global-gelatin-market-is-expected-to-reach-usd-279-billion-in-2018-transparency-market-research-213992871.html

[24] Kanmani P, Rhim JW. Physical, mechanical and antimicrobial properties of gelatin based active nanocomposite films containing AgNPs and nanoclay. Food Hydrocolloids. 2014;**35**:644-652

[25] Hosseini SF, Rezaei M, Zandi M, Farahmandghavi F. Development of bioactive fish gelatin/chitosan nanoparticles composite films with antimicrobial properties. Food Chemistry. 2016;**194**:1266-1274

[26] Uranga J, Puertas AI, Etxabide A, Duenas MT, Guerrero P, Caba KDL. Citric acid-incorporated fish gelatin/chitosan composite films. Food Hydrocolloids. 2018:1-9. In press. Available from: https://doi.org/10.1016/j.foodhyd.2018.02.018

[27] Oulkheir S, Ounine K, Haloui NEE, Attarassi B. Antimicrobial effect of citric, acetic, lactic acids and sodium nitrite against Escherichia Coli in tryptic soy broth. Journal of Biology, Agriculture and Healthcare. 2015;**5**(3):12-19

[28] Sarode AR, Sawale PD, Khedkar CD, Kalyankar SD, Pawshe RD. Casein and caseinate: Methods of manufacture. In: The Encyclopedia of Food and Health. Vol. 1. London, UK: Oxford, Academic Press; 2016. pp. 676-682

[29] Bonnaillie LM, Zhang H, Akkurt S, Yam KL, Tomasula PM. Casein films: The effects of formulation, environmental conditions and the addition of citric pectin on the structure and mechanical properties. Polymer. 2014;**6**:2018-2036

[30] Arrieta MP, Peltzer MA, López J, Garrigós MDC, Valente AJM, Jiménez A. Functional properties of sodium and calcium caseinate antimicrobial active films containing carvacrol. Journal of Food Engineering. 2013;**121**:94-101

[31] Broumand A, Djomeh ZE, Hamedi M, Razavi SH. Antimicrobial, water vapour permeability, mechanical and thermal properties of casein based zataraia multiflora boiss. Extract containing film. LWT–Food Science and Technology. 2011;**44**:2316-2323

[32] Oussalah M, Caillet S, Salmiéri S, Saucier L, Lacroix M. Antimicrobial and antioxidant effects of milk protein based film containing essential oils for the preservation of whole beef muscle. Journal of Agricultural and Food Chemistry. 2004;**52**(18):5598-5605

[33] Miladi H, Zmantar T, Chaabouni Y, Fedhila K, Bakhrouf A, Mahdouani K, et al. Antibacterial and efflux pump inhibitors of thymol and carvacrol against food-borne pathogens. Microbial Pathogenesis. 2016;**99**:95-100

[34] Research and Markets 2018. Global Whey Protein Market 2018 Analysis & Forecasts 2014-2022. Report. pp. 1-175

[35] Solak BB, Akin N. Functionality of whey protein. International Journal of Health and Nutrition. 2012;**3**(1):1-7

[36] Regalado C, Pérez-Pérez C, Lara-Cortés E, García-Almendarez B. Whey protein based edible food packaging films and coatings. Advances in Agricultural and Food Biotechnology. 2006:237-261

[37] Ribeiro-Santos R, Motta JFG, Teodoro CES, Melo NR. Antimicrobial effectiveness and color stability of protein-based films incorporated with essential oils. International Food Research Journal. 2017;**24**(5):2201-2206

[38] Seydim AC, Sarikus G. Antimicrobial activity of whey protein based edible films incorporated with oregano, rosemary and garlic essential oils. Food Research International. 2006;**39**:639-644

[39] Oliveira SPLF, Bertan LC, Rensis CMVBD, Bilck AP, Vianna PCB. Whey protein-based films incorporated with oregano essential oil. Polímeros. 2017;**27**(2):158-164

[40] Beristain-Bauza SDC, Mani-Lopez E, Palou E, Lopez-Malo A. Antimicrobial activity of whey protein films supplemented with *Lactobacillus sakei* cell-free supernatant on fresh beef. Food Microbiology. 2017;**62**:207-211

[41] Urso R, Cocolin L, Comi G. Cloning and sequencing of the Sakp operon from *Lactobacillus Sakei* isolated from naturally fermented sausages. In: Proceedings Book of the 19th International ICFMH Symposium Foodmicro. Portoroz, Slovenia; 2004;**157**:12-16

[42] Manab A, Sawitri ME, Al Awwaly KU, Purnomo H. Antimicrobial activity of whey protein based edible film incorporated with organic acids. African Journal of Food Science. 2011;**5**(1):6-11

[43] Anderson TJ, Lamsal BP. Zein extraction from corn, corn products, and coproducts and modifications for various applications: A review. Cereal Chemistry. 2011;**88**(2):159-173

[44] Informa Economics, Inc. A study assessing the opportunities and potential of corn-based products and technologies. Report for Agricultural Utilization Research Institute; 2009. p. 106

[45] Shukla R, Cheryan M. Zein: The industrial protein from corn. Industrial Crops and Products. 2001;**13**:171-192

[46] Moradi M, Tajik H, Rohani SMR, Mahmoudian A. Antioxidant and antimicrobial effects of zein edible film impregnated with *Zataria Multiflora* Boiss. Essential oil and monolaurin. LWT–Food Science and Technology. 2016;**72**:37-43

[47] Mei L, Teng Z, Zhu G, Liu Y, Zhang F, Zhang J, et al. Silver nanocluster-embedded zein films as antimicrobial coating materials for food packaging. ACS Applied Materials and Interfaces. 2017;**9**:35297-35304

[48] Ghiuta I, Cristeaa D, Croitorub C, Kost J, Wenkert R, Vyrides I, et al. Characterization and antimicrobial activity of silver nanoparticles, biosynthesized using bacillus species. Applied Surface Science. 2018;**438**:66-73

[49] Malhotra B, Keshwani A, Kharkwal H. Antimicrobial food packaging: Potential and pitfalls. Frontiers in Microbiology. 2015;**6**(611):1-9

[50] Deng X, Nikiforov AY, Leys C. Antimicrobial nanocomposites for food packaging. In: Nanotechnology in the Agri-food industry, Food Preservation. San Diego: Elsevier; 2017;**6**:1-34

[51] Shankar S, Jaiswal L, Rhim JW. Gelatin-based nanocomposite films: Potential use in antimicrobial active packaging. In: Antimicrobial Food Packaging. Academic Press, Elsevier; 2016. pp. 339-348

[52] Pisoschi AM, Pop A, Georgescu C, Turcus¸ V, Olah NK, Mathe E. An overview of natural antimicrobials role in food. European Journal of Medicinal Chemistry. 2018;**143**:922-935

[53] Seow YX, Yeo CR, Chung HL, Yuk HG. Plant essential oils as active antimicrobial agents. Critical Reviews in Food Science and Nutrition. 2014;**54**:625-644

[54] Yanwong S, Threepopnatkul P. Effect of peppermint and citronella essential oils on properties of fish skin gelatin edible films. IOP Conference Series: Materials Science and Engineering. 2015;**87**:012064

[55] Inouye S, Takizawa T, Yamaguchi H. Antibacterial activity of essential oils and their major constituents against respiratory tract pathogens by gaseous contact. Journal of Antimicrobial Chemotherapy. 2001;**47**(5):565-573

[56] Singh BR, Agrawal R, Prasanna V, Bhardwaj M, Dubey S. Antimicrobial activity of citronella essential oil on antimicrobial drug resistant bacteria from veterinary clinical cases. Clinical and Medical Biochemistry. 2015;**1**(106):1-9

[57] Martucci JF, Gende LB, Neira LM, Ruseckaite RA. Oregano and lavender essential oils as antioxidant and antimicrobial additives of biogenic gelatin films. Industrial Crops and Products. 2015;**71**:205-213

[58] Aisha I, Abdullahi Y. Development of whey protein concentrate edible membrane with cinnamon essential oil. Journal of Advances in Biology and Biotechnology. 2017;**11**(2):1-14

[59] Zhang Y, Liu X, Wang Y, Jiang P, Quek SY. Antibacterial activity and mechanism of cinnamon essential oil against *Escherichia Coli* and *Staphylococcus Aureus*. Food Control. 2016;**59**:282-289

[60] Hayek SA, Gyawali R, Ibrahim SA. Antimicrobial natural products. In: Microbial Pathogens and Strategies for Combating Them: Science, Technology and Education, Formatex Research Center.2013;**2**:910-921

[61] Kaewprachu P, Osako K, Benjakul S, Rawdkuen S. Quality attributes of minced pork wrapped with catechin–lysozyme incorporated gelatin film. Food Packaging and Shelf Life. 2015;**3**:88-96

[62] Malinowska-Pañczyk E, Staroszczyk H, Gottfried K, Kolodziejska I, Wojtasz-Pajak A. Antimicrobial properties of chitosan solutions, chitosan films and gelatin-chitosan films. Polimery. 2015;**60**:11-12

[63] Goy RC, Morais STB, Assis OBG. Evaluation of the antimicrobial activity of chitosan and its quaternized derivative on *E. Coli* and *S. Aureus*

growth. Revista Brasileira de Farmacognosia. 2016;**26**(1):122-127

[64] Lemire JA, Harrison JJ, Turner RJ. Antimicrobial activity of metals: Mechanisms, molecular targets and applications. Nature Reviews Microbiology. 2013;**11**(6):371-384

[65] Martucci JF, Ruseckaite RA. Antibacterial activity of gelatin/copper (II)-exchanged montmorillonite films. Food Hydrocolloids. 2017;**64**:70-77

[66] Divya M, Vaseeharan B, Abinaya M, Vijayakumar S, Govindarajan M, Alharbi NS, et al. Biopolymer gelatin-coated zinc oxide nanoparticles showed high antibacterial, antibiofilm and anti-angiogenic activity. Journal of Photochemistry and Photobiology, B: Biology. 2018;**178**:211-218

[67] Pasquet J, Chevalier Y, Couval E, Bouvier D, Noizet G, Morlière C, et al. Antimicrobial activity of zinc oxide particles on five micro-organisms of the challenge tests related to their physicochemical properties. International Journal of Pharmaceutics. 2014;**460**:92-100

[68] Sirelkhatim A, Mahmud S, Seeni A, Kaus AHM, Ann LC, Bakhori SKM, et al. Review on zinc oxide nanoparticles: Antibacterial activity and toxicity mechanism. Nano-Micro Letters. 2015;7(3):219-242

[69] Shankar S, Teng X, Li G, Rhim JW. Preparation, characterization, and antimicrobial activity of gelatin/Zno nanocomposite films. Food Hydrocolloids. 2015;**45**:264-271

[70] Dakal TC, Kumar A, Majumdar RS, Yadav V. Mechanistic basis of antimicrobial actions of silver nanoparticles. Frontiers in Microbiology. 2016;7:1831

[71] Kore VT, Tawade SS, Kabir J. Application of edible coatings on fruits and vegetables. Imperial Journal of Interdisciplinary Research. 2017;**3**(1):591-603

Chapter 5

Edible Films Incorporated with Active Compounds: Their Properties and Application

Saroat Rawdkuen

Abstract

Antimicrobial compounds are food additives, which play a major role to reduce food spoilage. There are three main groups of antimicrobial compounds such as chemical agent, natural extract, and probiotics. The direct incorporations of the active compounds on the surface of food may have limited benefit because they are rapidly diffused from the food surface into the food product, resulting in the limited efficacy of these compounds. Thus, incorporation of antimicrobial compounds into packaging matrix, especially biopolymer film is a promising technique to reduce contaminations and inhibit, retard, and/or kill the microorganisms. Edible films are thin layer of natural polymers used to maintain the physicochemical quality of foods and extend their shelf life. A variety of biopolymeric-based materials including polysaccharides, proteins, and lipids have been extensively used for antimicrobial packaging and can be used as a carrier of active compounds. Incorporation of antimicrobial compounds may or may not enhance the mechanical properties and water vapor permeability of biopolymer films. The applications of active films can reduce contamination through the releasing of antimicrobial compound, thus reducing the risk from pathogen, extending shelf life of the packaged foods, and providing better quality with high safety.

Keywords: antimicrobial, edible film, bioactive compounds, natural extract, shelf life extension

1. Introduction

Antimicrobial compounds are functional additives, which play a major role to reduce food spoilage, maintain quality, and increase the shelf life of foodstuffs. There are three main groups of antimicrobial compounds such as chemical agent, natural extracts, and probiotics. Recently, consumers are increasingly seeking foods containing natural-occurring substances rather than synthetic additive because some synthetic additives can promote carcinogenic and toxicity, which is a clear concern to the health of consumers [1]. The use of antimicrobial compounds by directly adding to food products may cause the reduction of active compounds' activity and may change the organoleptic properties of the foods due to the complexity of food components and strong flavor of some agents. Thus, the incorporation of antimicrobial compounds into packaging matrix is a promising technique that can increase antimicrobial efficiency and solve the limitation of directly adding.

A variety of biopolymeric-based materials including polysaccharides, proteins, and lipids have been frequently used as packaging materials. Currently, many researchers have focused on the inclusion of natural extracts such as catechin, lysozyme, *Careya sphaerica* Roxb., the extract of longan seed, coconut husk, and lemongrass essential oils in biopolymeric-based edible films [1–5]. Edible films exhibit various advantages such as edibility, non-toxicity, biodegradability, biocompatibility, and barrier properties against oxygen and physical stress [1, 2, 4, 5]. In this context, they serve as a carrier of antimicrobial substances to prevent the microbial spoilage of foods.

The qualities of foods, including appearance, color, and texture, are important attributes; those influence consumers' perception and satisfaction. Most of the foods are highly perishable due to their food components, which make them prone to microbial deterioration. In addition, the growth of microorganisms can accelerate food deterioration leading to undesirable flavor and odor, discoloration, and change in texture. Therefore, the application of antimicrobial biopolymer film may allow the release of antimicrobial agents with continued antimicrobial effect on the surface of foods during controlled condition storage. This chapter will review the recent research on the properties of antimicrobial biopolymer films and its application on various types of foodstuffs.

2. Antimicrobial compounds incorporated in the edible films

Antimicrobial compounds are additives used to control biological deterioration and to inhibit the growth of microorganisms, including pathogenic microorganisms. There are several groups of antimicrobial compounds potentially incorporated into edible films, including chemical agents, natural extracts, and probiotics. Most of the antimicrobial compounds are classified as generally recognized as safe (GRAS). Recently, the consumer's desire for natural substances and for chemical preservative-free foods has been continuously increased.

A wide variety of antimicrobial substances could be incorporated into a packaging material to enhance antimicrobial property for controlling the growth rate of specific or groups of microorganisms in headspace of the package, ensuring food safety, and extending product shelf life. Many antimicrobial agents have shown strong antimicrobial activity against target microorganisms in the culture media. Nevertheless, many antimicrobial agents have limited effect on the microorganisms, used as food additives. The selection of antimicrobial compounds for food packaging materials should be based on the nature of active agents and their inhibition mechanisms, physicochemical characteristics of foods and the organoleptic property of active compounds, packaging manufacturing process and their effect on the efficiency of active agents, storage conditions, toxicity and regulatory issues, microflora of foods and the physiology of target microorganisms, and releasing mechanisms of active substances into foods [6]. Thereafter, antimicrobial compounds will be classified according to their nature.

2.1 Chemical agents

Organic acids and their salts are generally used as chemical antimicrobial agents for food products due to their efficacy and cost. They are produced by chemical synthesis or chemical modification of natural acids [7]. They showed antimicrobial effects on many types of microorganisms and had been potentially incorporated into edible films. The commonly used organic acids in film packaging are acetic acid, lactic acid, sorbic acid, citric acid, and their salts. Many studies have developed organic acid-contained biopolymer films and reported their antimicrobial activity. For example, Uranga et al. [8] reported that 20% (w/w) citric acid-contained gelatin/chitosan films reduced *Escherichia coli* in liquid culture. da Rocha et al. [9] developed an anchovy protein films containing 1.50% (w/v) of sorbic acid or benzoic acid and evaluated antifungal effect of these films. The results suggested an effectiveness of antifungal films against *Aspergillus flavus* and *Rhizopus oryzae*. Organic acids can inhibit the growth of microorganisms by decreasing the pH, influencing the proton gradient cross membrane, acidifying the cytoplasm, and hindering transport chemicals across the cell membrane [10].

2.2 Natural extracts

2.2.1 Essential oils

Essential oils are aromatic and volatile oily extracts. Most of them are obtained from plant materials including leaves, flowers, roots, buds, and bark [11]. They can be utilized as flavoring in foodstuffs. However, the direct inclusion of essential oils as food preservatives is frequently limited owing to strong flavor. To avoid this problem, essential oils can be added into the edible films. The common used essential oils in bio-based film materials are cinnamon, clove, ginger, lemongrass, marjoram, oregano, sage, thyme, *Eucalyptus globulus*, and *Ziziphora clinopodioides*. They have shown to be against the various microorganisms [2, 12–15]. The antimicrobial activity of essential oils can be attributed to their major phenolic compounds such as thymol, eugenol, carvacrol, or terpenic compounds (α-pinene, β-pinene, 1,8-cineol, menthol, linalool), which are present in concentrations as much as 85% [11]. Different types of essential oils exhibited differences in their major compounds which had different ability to bind the membrane proteins of microbial cells and change the membrane permeability [16].

2.2.2 Plant and/or spice extracts

Recently, there has been an increasing interest in plants and/or spice extracts owing to the high levels of bioactive ingredients. Most of them are known to have a wide antimicrobial spectrum against microorganisms. The extracts can be obtained from various parts of plant and spice, including seeds, roots, bark, buds, flowers, and leaves. Antimicrobial efficiency of plant and/or spice extracts is generally attributed to the phenolic compounds that present in extracts. Phenolic compounds such as catechin, tannin, ferulic acid, caffeic acid, gallic acid, and carvacrol are present in parts of plants. Apart from antimicrobial efficiency, other benefits they offer include antioxidant capacity and their effect as alternative medicines. They are generally more effective against Gram-positive bacteria than that against Gram-negative bacteria due to the complex cell structure of Gram-negative bacteria.

2.2.3 Enzyme

The most employed as an antimicrobial enzyme is lysozyme. Lysozyme is a nutraceutical and is produced from egg white, milk, and blood [10]. It showed to be more effective against Gram-positive bacteria than Gram-negative bacteria by separating the bonds between N-acetylmuramic acid and N-acetylglucosamine of the peptidoglycan in the cell wall of bacteria [17]. Rawdkuen et al. [17] studied the antimicrobial effect of lysozyme on *Escherichia coli*, *Staphylococcus aureus*, *Listeria innocua*, and *Saccharomyces cerevisiae* and found that lysozyme could inhibit only the growth of *L. innocua* and *S. cerevisiae*. Furthermore, it has been reported that the combination of lysozyme with other substances can initiate membrane disruption. Rawdkuen et al. [17] found that the combination of lysozyme with catechin in the ratio of 1:1 showed significance inhibited in all microorganisms tested, when compared with lysozyme alone. Branen and Davidson [18] reported that small amounts of ethylenediamine tetraacetic acid (EDTA) could enhance the activity of lysozyme against Gram-negative bacteria. The use of antimicrobial enzyme should be considered carefully because antimicrobial efficiency is highly sensitive to the substrates and the environments. For instance, lysozyme activity can be significantly influenced by pH and temperature.

2.2.4 Bacteriocins

Bacteriocins are naturally occurring antimicrobial substances. They are small molecular weight peptides produced by microorganisms and effectively inhibit the growth of food spoilage bacteria, mainly Gram-positive bacteria [10]. Many bacteriocins, including nisin, pediocin, and lacticin, can be incorporated into edible films to inhibit the growth of spoilage and pathogenic microorganisms. The most employed as antimicrobial bacteriocins is nisin. Nisin is an antimicrobial peptide which is produced by *Lactococcus lactis* ssp. *Lactis* and is known to exhibit antimicrobial activity against a wide range of Gram-positive bacteria. It has limited activity against Gram-negative bacteria because of its inability to penetrate the cell and reach to the cytoplasmic membrane [10]. Many studies have been reported that the combination of nisin with chelating agent (EDTA) improves the antimicrobial activity of nisin against Gram-negative bacteria by destabilizing the outer membrane and then releasing the lipopolysaccharide layer and allowing nisin to access the cytoplasmic membrane [19–21]. Antimicrobial efficiency of bacteriocins is influenced by its concentrations and number and species of microorganisms, using condition, interaction or inactivation by food elements, and temperature and pH of product [10].

2.3 Probiotics

Probiotics are live microorganisms that have a beneficial effect on health upon ingestion in sufficient numbers [22]. The most frequently used bacteria belong to the genera *Lactobacillus* and *Bifidobacterium*, although *Streptococcus thermophilus* and *Saccharomyces boulardii* are available in some dairy products. These naturally produced antimicrobial can inhibit the growth of strains of other bacteria. The use of probiotics can efficiently control the competitive undesirable microorganisms [7]. Recently, Bekhit et al. [23] reported that hydroxypropyl methylcellulose (HPMC) films containing microencapsulation of *Lactococcus lactis* subsp. *Lactis* showed effectiveness to reduce the growth of *L. monocytogenes* by five-log cycle after 12 days of storage, compared to the control film (without addition of *L. lactis*). Beristain-Bauza et al. [24] reported that whey protein isolate films containing cell-free supernatant of *L. rhamnosus* (12 or 18 mg/ml to film-forming solution) showed inhibitory activity against Gram-negative (*E. coli* and *Salmonella typhimurium*) and Gram-positive bacteria (*L. monocytogenes* and *S. aureus*). In addition, probiotics may be carried within edible polymer matrix used in the food packaging industry due to its safety and effectiveness.

3. Properties of biopolymer-based film

Antimicrobial film should be provided the same basic functions as the traditional food packaging. In general, the properties of edible film depend on type of raw material, film additive, concentration, process for making film, and condition used [25]. All of these factors must also be taken into account when making antimicrobial biopolymer-based film. When antimicrobial substance is incorporated into edible film to retard the microbial growth, it can adversely change the original mechanical integrity, barrier properties, physical properties, and thermal stability of edible film. General properties of edible film include mechanical properties (tensile strength and elongation at break), barrier properties (water vapor permeability), and optical properties (color and transparency).

3.1 Mechanical properties

Mechanical properties are basic functions of food packaging which protect the food from physical damage such as denting, breaking, and bruising. The investigation of mechanical properties of antimicrobial film can provide the information of the film flexibility and the resistance of the film to the force. This information will be also used to predict the efficiency of antimicrobial film during handling, storage, or use. Mechanical properties are commonly expressed as tensile strength (TS) and elongation at break (EAB). TS represents the maximum strength that a film can withstand, while EAB is the measurement of the ability of a film to stretch. The mechanical properties of antimicrobial bio-based film are shown in **Table 1**.

Incorporation of antimicrobial compounds may or may not enhance the mechanical properties of edible films. It has been frequently reported that the mechanical properties of antimicrobial film are strongly dependent on concentration of antimicrobial compounds. Higher concentrations of antimicrobial agent are expected to lead to lower film strength and greater film extensibility because high amounts of antimicrobial compound inclusion may help to enhance the plasticizing effect of the edible film, as a consequence improving the film's extensibility [4, 5].

However, some researchers have reported that the inclusion of antimicrobial agent above a certain limit led to a decrease in the film stretch [1, 26]. Thus, prior to making antimicrobial film, the concentration of antimicrobial agent should be considered. Good mechanical properties are among the basic requirements for antimicrobial film to be used as active food packaging, since poor extensibility or strength may lead to premature failure or cracking during production, handling, storage, or use.

3.2 Barrier property

The barrier property extensively studied in food packaging material is water vapor permeability (WVP). WVP of packaging films is extremely the main function for preserving the quality or prolonging the shelf life of packaged food products. Generally, lower WVP values indicate decreasing film permeability, due to physiochemical deterioration and microbial spoilage that are related to the equilibrium moisture content. Thus, the film should have low WVP because the film is mainly used to avoid moisture transfer between the food and the environmental surrounding, as a result, maintaining quality and extending shelf life of packaged food products. However, the specific requirement for the films' WVP depends on characteristics of food products and intent use. **Table 1** summarizes data on WVP of various antimicrobial films.

It has been reported that the addition of antimicrobial agent into edible film could reduce the films' WVP has been reported. Antimicrobial films showed less WVP values than the films without addition of antimicrobial agents by about one–two times (**Table 1**). The dramatic decrease in the antimicrobial films' WVP is due to reduction in free volume space of polymer, decreasing an ability to bind with water molecules and increasing tortuosity of diffusive pathway through the film [1, 17, 27, 32]. However, antimicrobial substance-added edible films could also lead to higher in the films' WVP [3, 32]. It has been reported that antimicrobial agents could play

Based film	Antimicrobial compounds	Loading	Mechanical properties		WVP ($\times 10^{-10}$ g m/ m^2 s Pa)	Refs.
			TS (MPa)	EAB (%)		
Basil seed gum	Oregano essential oil	1–6% (v/v)	—	—	0.37–0.43	[27]
Chitosan	Apple peel polyphenols	0, 0.25, 0.50, 0.75, and 1%	16–27	13–28	1.00–1.47	[28]
Chitosan	Curcumin	0–1% (w/w, based on chitosan)	6.64–11.82	79.13–39.41	2.24–2.69	[29]
Chitosan	Turmeric extract	1:2 (v/v, chitosan: extract)	32.2–47.9	6.20–6.35	1.12–1.53	[30]
Sodium alginate	Sage oil	0–1% (v/v)	4.8–5.2	4–78	1.90–2.36	[16]
Sodium alginate-carboxymethyl cellulose	Cinnamon essential oil	5, 10, and 15% (w/v)	16.07–32.10	20.07–32.67	13.66–28.01	[31]
Tapioca starch	Grape pomace extracts	8% (v/v)	2.58–3.55	22.5–45.8	13.42–20.22	[32]
Chicken feet protein	Marjoram oil	0–1% (w/v)	7.13–7.59	11.92–21.78	25.90–34.90	[14]
Fish myofibrillar protein	Catechin-Kradon extract	0–12 mg/ml	6.53–10.31	51.38–132.76	15.60–20.80	[1]
Gelatin	Catechin-lysozyme	0–0.5% (w/v)	3.31–33.49	27.82–143.87	650–1360	[4]
Gelatin	Longan seed extract	50–500 ppm	49.53–52.84	17.42–18.62	0.29–0.40	[5]
Gelatin	Coconut husk extract	0–0.4% (w/w)	34.97–41.93	6.16–7.90	0.23–0.28	[3]

Table 1.
Mechanical properties and water vapor permeability (WVP) of antimicrobial films.

a role as a plasticizing agent in the films, leading to the interaction between intermolecular reduction and the enhancement of macromolecules' mobility [32]. As a consequence, the film had high WVP values. In addition, the films' WVP are affected by the chemical nature of macromolecules and additives, hydrophilic/hydrophobic ratios of the films, and the structural characteristic of macromolecules [32, 33].

3.3 Optical properties

Optical properties (color attributes and transparency) of food packaging are crucial parameters, which directly affect to the consumer acceptability and impact on product appearance. In general, color attributes are expressed as L* (lightness/darkness), a* (redness/greenness), and b* (yellowness/blueness) values. Transparency was used to evaluate film transparency wherein higher transparency value indicates lower film transparency. The optical properties of antimicrobial film packaging are summarized in **Table 2**. Recently, several researchers have reported that the addition of antimicrobial compounds could influence the optical properties of edible film by decreasing lightness and film transparency values and increasing redness and yellowness values correlated with the increasing content of antimicrobial agent [1, 5, 28].

Kaewprachu et al. [1] reported that the incorporation of catechin (obtained from commercial product)-Kradon extract (extracted from the leaves of *Careya sphaerica* Roxb.) could adversely affect the films' color, especially at higher amounts of catechin-Kradon extract. They concluded that the presence of natural pigment in catechin-Kradon extract can contribute to the color of fish myofibrillar protein film. Xu et al. [32] studied the effect of source of grape pomace extracts from Cabernet Franc (red variety) and Viognier (white variety) on the optical property of tapioca starch film. The results showed that source of extract had significant influence on film transparency. Inclusion of these extracts decreased transparency of films. Changes in films' color and transparency depend on source of active compounds, level of active agent incorporation, and original pigment present in active agent.

Therefore, film with low transparency may not be suitable for food packaging applications when the film is used as a see-through packaging material and used to enhance product's appearance. Although the color and transparency of antimicrobial film could affect the consumer perception, there are many advantages to helping to protect the packaged foods from ultraviolet and visible light that lead to discoloration, nutrient losses, and off-flavor and to showing antimicrobial properties that do not exist in the traditional packaging.

3.4 Antimicrobial property

The addition of antimicrobial compounds into edible films is expected to enhance their antimicrobial activity. Edible films can act as carriers of antimicrobial agents, which may either be immobilized into the film matrix or play their role upon contact with food surface or be slowly released into foodstuffs. The antimicrobial activity of films is commonly assessed through agar disc diffusion method, regarding the diffusion of substances tested through water-containing agar plate. The film cuts are placed on an agar surface which is previously inoculated with the test microorganisms, incubated under suitable conditions depending on the test microorganisms, and then observed the inhibition zone around the disc films [30]. The antimicrobial activity of antimicrobial agent-contained edible films was found against a wide variety of microorganisms, including bacteria and some fungi. The antimicrobial activity of active agents used in edible films against some microorganisms is presented in **Table 3**.

It has been frequently reported that inclusion of antimicrobial compounds has greatly enhanced antimicrobial property of edible films. Higher amounts of antimicrobial agent are expected to lead to higher antimicrobial effects. It should be noted that the antimicrobial efficiency of antimicrobial substances added into edible film can depend on the target microorganisms (Gram-positive bacteria, Gram-negative bacteria, fungi, and others), the type of antimicrobial agents, the level of antimicrobial agent incorporation, and their major compounds [14]. Most of the antimicrobial films showed more effectiveness against Gram-positive bacteria than Gram-negative bacteria. This is due to the cell wall lipopolysaccharides or the protection of outer membranes of Gram-negative bacteria which could inhibit the diffusion of antimicrobial agent into the cell, thus decreasing the microbial growth inhibition [31].

Based film	Antimicrobial compounds	Loading	Color attributes			Transparency	Refs.
			L^*	a^*	b^*		
Chitosan	Curcumin	0 and 1% (w/w, based on chitosan)	56.24–65.28	(−0.87)–8.17	5.54–47.56	1.36–2.12	[29]
Chitosan	Apple peel polyphenols	0, 0.25, 0.50, 0.75, and 1%	45.52–82.82	(−2.11)–29.17	8.12–47.76	0.71–4.28	[28]
Chitosan	*Ziziphora clinopodioides* essential oil	0 and 1% (v/w)	84.85–88.66	(−0.12)–(−1.76)	28.15–29.12	—	[34]
Tapioca starch	Grape pomace extracts	0 and 8% (v/v)	73.5–91.5	(−0.32)–10.8	3.91–15.2	0.38–0.60	[32]
Fish myofibrillar protein	Catechin-Kradon extract	0–12 mg/ml	88.92–95.01	(−0.68)–4.84	4.70–18.10	3.35–3.88	[1]
Gelatin	Longan seed extract	50–500 ppm	83.86–89.57	(−0.89)–(−2.20)	11.72–26.43	3.24–3.36	[5]
Gelatin	Grape seed extract	0 and 1% (v/w)	55.12–91.42	(−2.51)–16.77	12.57–15.81	—	[34]

Table 2.
Color attributes and transparency of edible films incorporated with antimicrobial compounds.

DOI: http://dx.doi.org/10.5772/intechopen.80707

Based film	Antimicrobial compounds	Loading	Microorganism(s) tested	Results	Refs.
Chitosan	Curcumin	1% (w/w, based on chitosan)	*S. aureus* and *R. solani*	Microorganisms exhibited sensitivity to antimicrobial films	[29]
Chitosan	Propolis extract	2.5–20% (w/w)	*S. aureus*, *S. enteritidis*, *E. coli*, and *P. aeruginosa*	Inhibiting all bacteria tested on contact surface	[35]
Chitosan	Turmeric extract	1:2 (v/v, chitosan: extract ratio)	*S. aureus* and *Salmonella*	Reduced the count of bacteria tested	[30]
Corn starch-beeswax	Lauric arginate+ natamycin	2000 mg/l + 400 mg/l	*R. stolonifer*, *C. gloeosporioides*, *B. cinerea*, and *S.* Saintpaul	Completely inhibited all microorganisms tested	[38]
Tapioca starch	Grape pomace extracts	8% (v/v)	*S. aureus* and *L. monocytogenes*	Exhibited a stronger inhibitory effect on *S. aureus* compared to *L. monocytogenes*	[32]
Chicken feet protein	Marjoram oil	1% (w/v)	*E. coli* O157:H7, *S.* enteritidis, *L. monocytogenes*, and *S. aureus*	Inhibited all bacteria tested	[14]
Gelatin	Lemongrass oil	5–25% (w/w based on protein)	*E. coli*, *L. monocytogenes*, *S. aureus*, and *S. typhimurium*	Inhibited all bacteria tested	[2]
Gelatin	Grape seed extract + *Ziziphora clinopodioides* essential oil	1% (v/w) + 1% (v/w)	*S. aureus*, *B. subtilis*, *B. cereus*, *L. monocytogenes*, *S. typhimurium*, and *E. coli*	Effectively against Gram-positive bacteria	[34]
Fish myofibrillar protein	Catechin-Kradon extract	3–12 mg/ml	*S. aureus*, *E. coli*, *S. typhimurium*, and *V. parahaemolyticus*	They showed microbial inhibitory effects on the contact surface against all bacteria tested	[1]
Whey protein	Rosemary and thyme extracts	3 and 5%	*L. monocytogenes* and *S. aureus*	Inhibited all bacteria tested	[39]

Table 3.
Antimicrobial activity of some compounds used in edible films against some microorganisms.

However, some studies have reported that edible films incorporated with antimicrobial substance did not show any antimicrobial effect on microorganisms. Siripatrawan and Vitchayakitti [35] observed that chitosan films containing propolis extract at different concentrations (2.5–20%, w/w based on chitosan content) did not show any inhibition zone, but they could inhibit bacteria tested on contact surface. They concluded that chitosan polymer and phenolic compounds that present in propolis extract are tightly interacted and led to reduce the release or diffusion of antimicrobial substances from the chitosan film matrix to inhibit bacteria surrounding film disc during agar disc diffusion method.

In addition, the diffusion or releasing of antimicrobial substance through the film is also affected by the composition, manufacturing method, hydrophilic-hydrophobic balance of the antimicrobial agent, and storage conditions [7]. Furthermore, the performance of antimicrobial compounds against the specific or groups of microorganisms and the different interactions among the biopolymer material, the antimicrobial substance, and presented food components also affect this phenomenon [36]. All of these factors can be altered, the antimicrobial activity and the edible films' properties. Therefore, these are being key factors for the making of antimicrobial films.

4. Applications of antimicrobial biopolymer-based film

Appearance, color, and texture are crucial factors that consumers will consider prior to making a decision to buy fresh produce and meat products. Most foods are highly perishable due to their biological and chemical compositions. Pathogen contamination or food deterioration usually occurs on the food surface. When this phenomenon occurred, the food showed undesirable odors and visible changes on the surface of foods. The growth of microorganisms is the most problem of food spoilage which can lower quality and decrease the shelf life and changes in natural microflora that could induce pathogenic problems. Furthermore, microbial growth in foods also significantly reduces the safety of food and the security of public health. Microbial spoilage of foodstuffs is caused by many species of microorganisms, including bacteria, yeast, and molds. However, the food spoilage by microorganisms is dependent upon pH, water activity, nutrients, and presence of oxygen [7].

Various food processing technologies have been developed to prevent the contamination and to inactivate the pathogenic microorganisms. Many nonthermal processing technologies, such as irradiation, high-pressure process, and pulsed electric field, are being studied to estimate their mechanisms and effectiveness in microbial inhibition. However, these technologies may not completely prevent or control pathogenic microorganisms due to the complexity of food composition, a wide variety of microbial physiology, passage of contamination, pathogenic mechanisms, and the mass-production nature of food processing [7]. The use of antimicrobial compounds also reduces or inhibits the microbial population that present in the foods.

The direct inclusion of antimicrobial agents to food products can reduce the antimicrobial activity of antimicrobial compounds because the food components can interfere or reduce their efficiency. Furthermore, some antimicrobial compounds exhibit strong flavor/color which may change the organoleptic properties of food products. Therefore, the antimicrobial film is a promising way to slowly migrate the antimicrobial compound to the surface of foods and enable continued antimicrobial effect on the food surface during extended storage, which may act as additional hurdles against food spoilage. This polymer-based film system can be applied to various types of food products such as meat, seafood, fruits, and vegetables, in order to maintain quality, enhance food safety, and prolong the shelf life of foods.

In recent years, the applications of antimicrobial films on the real food system were reported. For instance, Putsakum et al. [40] developed 0.3% (w/v) of neem extract (*Azadirachta indica*)-contained gelatin films, applied on minced beef, and determined the quality of minced beef during storage 4 ± 1°C for 7 days (**Figure 1A**). The results showed that minced beef wrapped with gelatin films containing Neem extract had lower in TBARS value than the sample wrapped with polyvinyl chloride (PVC). Kaewprachu et al. [41] suggested that fish myofibrillar protein films incorporated with 9 mg/ml of catechin-Kradon extract could delay discoloration, lipid oxidation, and the growth of microorganisms throughout the duration of storage (at 4 ± 1°C for 10 days) (**Figure 1B**).

4.1 Meat and meat-based products

Most of the fresh meat products are highly perishable due to their biological compositions. Fresh meat is generally composed of 12–20% of protein, 0–6% carbohydrates, and 3–45% fat, In fact, muscle tissue is made up of approximately 75.5% water, but this level can range from 42 to 80% [42]. Additionally, the presence of water in meat also affords microorganisms to support their growth. To reduce the growth and spread of pathogenic and spoilage microorganisms in meat foodstuffs, antimicrobial films can be used to inhibit, retard, or kill the growth of microorganisms. Similarly, antimicrobial packaging that releases antimicrobial agents also offers potential for reducing the effect of the growth of slime-forming bacteria on meat surface. Current applications of antimicrobial film on meat and meat-based products are summarized in **Table 4**.

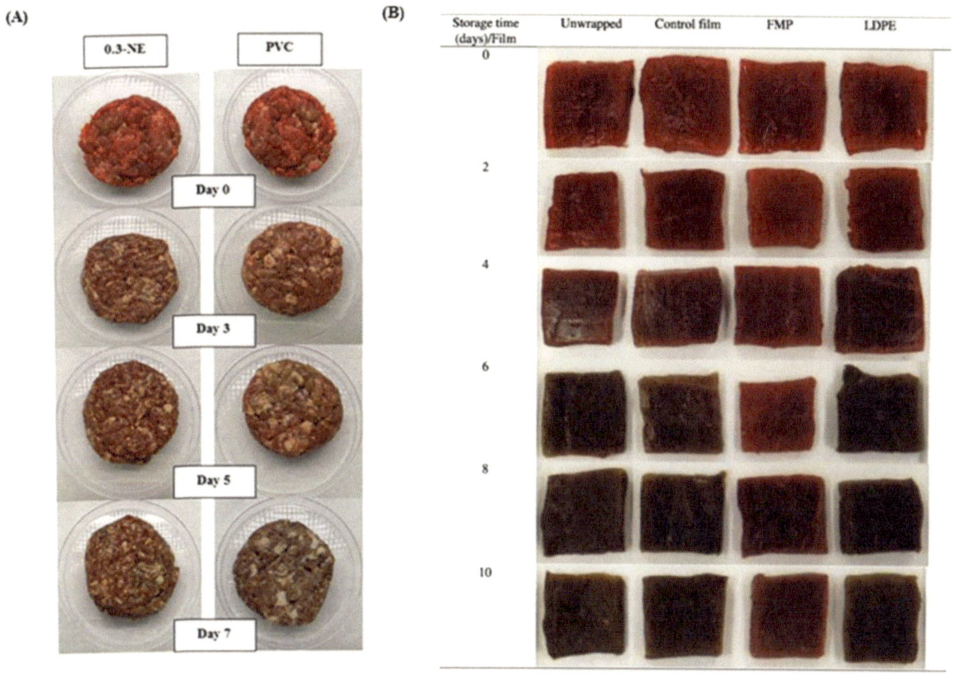

Figure 1.
Applications of gelatin films incorporated with 0.3% (w/v) of neem extract (NE) on minced beef during storage at 4 ± 1°C for 7 days (A) and fish myofibrillar protein (FMP) containing 9 mg/ml of catechin-Kradon extract on bluefin tuna flesh during storage at 4 ± 1°C for 10 days (B) compared with the commercial wrap films (PVC, polyvinyl chloride and LDPE, low density polyethylene) [40, 41].

Test substrates	Based film	Antimicrobial compounds	Concentration	Results	Refs.
Beef	Whey protein-sodium alginate	Rehydrated supernatant of *Lactobacillus sakei*	18 mg/ml	Reduced the population of *E. coli* by 2.3 log CFU/g after 36 h	[43]
Camel meat	Carboxymethyl cellulose	*Ziziphora clinopodioides* essential oil + *Ficus carica* extract	2% (v/v) + 1% (w/v)	Reduced the population of spoilage and pathogenic microorganisms	[44]
Chicken meat	Tapioca starch	Grape pomace extracts + cellulose nanocrystal	8% (v/v) + 10% (v/v)	Reduced the growth of *L. monocytogenes* by 1–2 log CFU/g during 10 days storage	[30]
Chicken fillets	Sodium alginate-galbanum gum	*Ziziphora persica* essential oils	0.5 and 1.0% (w/v)	Inhibition of natural microflora and *Pseudomonas* spp. of the chicken fillets	[46]
Ground beef	Cassava starch	Oregano essential oil + pumpkin residue extract	2% (w/v) + 3% (w/v)	Delayed the growth of coliform and *Salmonella*	[47]
Minced pork	Gelatin	Catechin-lysozyme	0.5% (w/v)	Inhibition of natural microflora of the minced pork	[48]
Pork sausage	Collagen	Nisin	10,000 ppm	Reduced the growth of *L. monocytogenes* by 1.1 log CFU/g	[49]
Sausage	Calcium alginate	*Terminalia arjuna* extract	0.5 and 1.0% (w/w)	Inhibition of natural microflora of the sausage	[50]
Ready to cook pork chops	Chitosan	Bamboo vinegar	2% (w/v)	Inhibiting microbial growth against total viable count, lactic acid bacteria, and *Pseudomonas* spp.	[51]

Table 4.
Application of antimicrobial films on meat and meat-based products.

4.2 Seafood-based products

Seafood products are highly perishable. Different categories of seafood products have unique spoilage patterns based upon innate compositional, chemical biochemical, and microbiological differences [22]. The growth of microorganisms can shorten the shelf life of seafood products by changing the organoleptic properties that affect consumers' acceptability of the products. Also, seafood-associated foodborne pathogen outbreaks are concern. Most of them are commonly contaminated with several pathogenic microorganisms such as *Vibrio parahaemolyticus*, *Escherichia coli*, *Salmonella*, and *Listeria monocytogenes*; however, others such as *Clostridium botulinum* and *Aeromonas hydrophila* are also associated with marine food products [52, 53]. Consumption of the contaminated seafood with pathogenic microorganisms can lead to foodborne illnesses in the form of infection, intoxication, or both [53]. Yücel and Balci [54] evaluated 78 fish samples (30 freshwater and 48 marine fish) for the presence of *Listeria* and *Aeromonas* species from fish market in Ankara, Turkey. The incidence of *Listeria* spp. was 30% in freshwater and 10.4%

Test substrates	Based film	Antimicrobial compounds	Concentration	Results	Refs.
Cold-smoked salmon	Gelatin	Olive leaf extract	5.63% (w/w)	Reduced the growth rate of *L. monocytogenes*	[52]
Deepwater pink shrimp	Chitosan	Orange essential oil	2% (v/v)	Inhibition of natural microflora of shrimp	[56]
Fish steak	Chitosan	Ginger essential oil	0.3% (v/v)	Inhibition of lactic acid bacteria and *B. thermosphacta*	[57]
Hake fillets	Whey protein isolate	Oregano and thyme essential oil	1 and 3% (w/w)	Reduction in psychrotrophic bacteria, H_2S-producing bacteria, and *Pseudomonas*	[58]
Shrimp	Gelatin	*Ziziphora clinopodioides* essential oil + pomegranate peel extract	1% (v/v)	Inhibition of *Pseudomonas* spp., *P. fluorescens*, *S. putrefaciens*, *Enterobacteriaceae*, and *L. monocytogenes*	[59]
Shrimp	Chitosan	Pomegranate peel extract	1.5% (w/v)	Inhibition of natural microbiota of shrimp	[60]
Sea bass slices	Fish protein isolate/ gelatin	Basil leaf essential oil	100% (w/w, based on protein)	Retarded microbial growth	[61]
Salmon	Barley bran protein/ gelatin	Grapefruit seed extract	1% (w/v)	Reduced the populations of *E. coli* O157:H7 and *L. monocytogenes*	[62]
Tuna slices	Fish myofibrillar protein	Catechin-Kradon extract	9 mg/ml	Inhibiting the growth of microorganisms	[41]
Fatty tuna meat	Red pepper seed meal protein/ gelatin	Oregano oil	0.5% (w/v)	Reduced the growth of *L. monocytogenes* and *S. typhimurium*	[63]

Table 5.
Application of antimicrobial films on seafood-based products.

Test substrates	Based coating	Active compounds	Concentration	Results	Refs.
Apple	Chitosan	Olive oil residue extract	20 g/l	Delayed the growth of *P. expansum* and *R. stolonifer* during cold storage (35 days)	[65]
Apple	Pullulan	*Satureja hortensis* extract	2, 5, 10, and 20% (w/v)	Reduced the growth of *S. aureus* by 1.4 log CFU/g (at 16°C for 21 days)	[66]
Arbutus berries	Alginate	Eugenol	0.2% (w/v)	Reduced microbial spoilage and arbutus berries can be stored for at least 28 days at 0.5 °C	[67]
Black radish	Chitosan-gelatin	Thyme essential oil	0.2%	Reduction the growth of *L. monocytogenes* by 2.1 log CFU/g after 24 h	[68]
Lime	Soy protein	Limonene	5 and 10% (w/w, based on protein)	Reduced wounds with *Penicillium italicum* by 85% after storage at 13°C for 13 days	[69]
Pepper	Pullulan	*Satureja hortensis* extract	2, 5, 10, and 20% (w/v)	Reduced the growth of *A. niger* by 1.33 log CFU/g (at 16°C for 21 days)	[65]
Strawberry	Chitosan	Olive oil residue extract	20 g/L	Delayed the growth of *P. expansum* and *R. stolonifer* during cold storage (16 days)	[66]
Strawberry	*Aloe vera*	Ascorbic acid	1, 3, and 5% (w/v)	Reducing microbial populations	[70]

Table 6.
Application of antimicrobial films on fresh and minimally processed fruits and vegetables.

in marine fish samples, while *Aeromonas* spp. isolated from marine fish samples (93.7%) showed higher than freshwater fish (10%), mainly *A. hydrophila*. They also reported that *Aeromonas* spp. can be primary or secondary pathogens of fish. Kahraman et al. [55] reported that the incidence of *A. hydrophila* and *Plesiomonas shigelloides* in 700 seafoods (400 fish, 100 shrimps, and 200 mollusks) was detected in 5.71 and 0.86%, respectively. Thus, the use of antimicrobial film could inhibit the microbial growth, preserve the quality, and prolong the shelf life of seafood. Current applications of antimicrobial packaging on seafood-based products are summarized in **Table 5**.

4.3 Fresh and minimally processed fruits and vegetables

Fruits and vegetables are classified as perishable products. They are very susceptible to biochemical, nutritional, and structural with textural changes. These postharvest changes can be accelerated by loss of water and microorganisms' action. Fungal are mostly associated microorganism outbreak that reduced the quality of fruits and vegetables [64]. The use of antimicrobial films and/or coatings could minimize the undesirable changes in fruit and vegetable; thus, the products have good quality, attractive organoleptic properties, and close to fresh product during extended storage. Current applications of antimicrobial packaging on fresh and minimally processed fruits and vegetables are summarized in **Table 6**.

5. Conclusions

There are many types of antimicrobial agents that could be incorporated into food packaging materials, especially bio-based films. The suitable selection of antimicrobial substances is crucial to obtain antimicrobial effectiveness. Antimicrobial film is a promising category of active packaging system which able to inhibit the growth of microorganisms and retard the developments of discoloration and off-flavors in food products. The addition of antimicrobial compounds into biopolymer-based edible films could improve the mechanical, water barrier, and antimicrobial properties. Most foods are perishable and are susceptible to microbial contamination. The use of antimicrobial films has shown to preserve quality and increase the shelf life of various food products. The enhancement in the quality of the food products is achieved through inhibiting the target microorganisms.

Acknowledgements

The author would like to thank the Mae Fah Luang University for the financial support. Dr. Pimonpan Kaewprachu was also acknowledged for the preparation of the whole parts of this manuscript and the revision.

Author details

Saroat Rawdkuen
Unit of Innovative Food Packaging and Biomaterials, School of Agro-Industry, Mae Fah Luang University, Chiang Rai, Thailand

*Address all correspondence to: saroat@mfu.ac.th

References

[1] Kaewprachu P, Rungraeng N, Osako K, Rawdkuen S. Properties of fish myofibrillar protein film incorporated with catechin-Kradon extract. Food Packaging and Shelf Life. 2017;**13**:56-65. DOI: 10.1016/j.fpsl.2017.07.003

[2] Ahmad M, Benjakul S, Prodpran T, Agustini T. Physico-mechanical and antimicrobial properties of gelatin film from the skin of unicorn leatherjacket incorporated with essential oils. Food Hydrocolloids. 2012;**28**:189-199. DOI: 10.1016/j.foodhyd.2011.12.003

[3] Nagarajan M, Benjakul S, Prodpran T, Songtipya P. Properties and characteristics of nanocomposite films from tilapia skin gelatin incorporated with ethanolic extract from coconut husk. Journal of Food Science and Technology. 2015;**52**:7669-7682. DOI: 10.1007/s13197-015-1905-1

[4] Rawdkuen S, Suthiluk P, Kamhangwong D, Benjakul S. Mechanical, physico-chemical, and antimicrobial properties of gelatin-based film incorporated with catechin-lysozyme. Chemistry Central Journal. 2012;**6**:131. DOI: 10.1186/1752-153X-6-131

[5] Vichasilp C, Sai-Ut S, Benjakul S, Rawdkuen S. Effect of longan seed extract and BHT on physical and chemical properties of gelatin based film. Food Biophysics. 2014;**9**:238-248. DOI: 10.1007/s11483-014-9345-4

[6] Coma V. Antimicrobial and antioxidant active packaging for meat and poultry. In: Kerry JP, editor. Advances in Meat, Poultry and Seafood Packaging. Cambridge: Woodhead Publishing; 2012. pp. 477-498

[7] Han JH. Antimicrobial packaging systems. In: Han JH, editor. Innovations in Food Packaging. London: Elsevier Science; 2005. pp. 80-101

[8] Uranga J, Puertas AI, Etxabide A, Dueñas MT, Guerrero P, de la Caba K. Citric acid-incorporated fish gelatin/chitosan composite films. Food Hydrocolloids. 2019;**86**:95-103. DOI: 10.1016/j.foodhyd.2018.02.018

[9] da Rocha M, Prietto L, de Souza MM, Furlong EB, Prentice C. Effect of organic acids on physical-mechanical and antifungicidal properties of anchovy protein films. Journal of Aquatic Food Product Technology. 2018;**27**:316-326. DOI: 10.1080/10498850.2018.1433736

[10] Naidu AS. Overview. In: Naidu AS, editor. Natural Food Antimicrobial Systems. London: CRC Press; 2000. pp. 1-16

[11] Burt S. Essential oils: Their antibacterial properties and potential applications in foods—A review. International Journal of Food Microbiology. 2004;**94**:223-253. DOI: 10.1016/j.ijfoodmicro.2004.03.022

[12] Ejaz M, Arfat YA, Mulla M, Ahmed J. Zinc oxide nanorods/clove essential oil incorporated Type B gelatin composite films and its applicability for shrimp packaging. Food Packaging and Shelf Life. 2018;**15**:113-121. DOI: 10.1016/j.fpsl.2017.12.004

[13] Hafsa J, Ma S, Ben Khedher MR, Charfeddine B, Limem K, Majdoub H, et al. Physical, antioxidant and antimicrobial properties of chitosan films containing *Eucalyptus globulus* essential oil. LWT—Food Science and Technology. 2016;**68**:356-364. DOI: 10.1016/j.lwt.2015.12.050

[14] Lee J-H, Lee J, Song KB. Development of a chicken feet protein film containing essential oils. Food Hydrocolloids. 2015;**46**:208-215. DOI: 10.1016/j.foodhyd.2014.12.020

[15] Martucci JF, Gende LB, Neira LM, Ruseckaite RA. Oregano and lavender essential oils as antioxidant and antimicrobial additives of biogenic gelatin films. Industrial Crops and Products. 2015;**71**:205-213. DOI: 10.1016/j.indcrop.2015.03.079

[16] Acevedo-Fani A, Salvia-Trujillo L, Rojas-Graü MA, Martín-Belloso O. Edible films from essential-oil-loaded nanoemulsions: Physicochemical characterization and antimicrobial properties. Food Hydrocolloids. 2015;**47**:168-177. DOI: 10.1016/j.foodhyd.2015.01.032

[17] Rawdkuen S, Suthiluk P, Kamhangwong D, Benjakul S. Antimicrobial activity of some potential active compounds against food spoilage microorganisms. African Journal of Biotechnology. 2012;**11**:13914-13921. DOI: 10.5897/AJB12.1400

[18] Branen JK, Davidson PM. Enhancement of nisin, lysozyme, and monolaurin antimicrobial activities by ethylenediaminetetraacetic acid and lactoferrin. International Journal of Food Microbiology. 2004;**90**:63-74. DOI: 10.1016/S0168-1605(03)00172-7

[19] Prudêncio CV, Mantovani HC, Cecon PR, Prieto M, Vanetti MCD. Temperature and pH influence the susceptibility of *Salmonella typhimurium* to nisin combined with EDTA. Food Control. 2016;**61**:248-253. DOI: 10.1016/j.foodcont.2015.09.042

[20] Morsy MK, Elsabagh R, Trinetta V. Evaluation of novel synergistic antimicrobial activity of nisin, lysozyme, EDTA nanoparticles, and/or ZnO nanoparticles to control foodborne pathogens on minced beef. Food Control. 2018;**92**:249-254. DOI: 10.1016/j.foodcont.2018.04.061

[21] Sivarooban T, Hettiarachchy NS, Johnson MG. Physical and antimicrobial properties of grape seed extract, nisin, and EDTA incorporated soy protein edible films. Food Research International. 2008;**41**:781-785. DOI: 10.1016/j.foodres.2008.04.007

[22] Dehghani S, Hosseini SV, Regenstein JM. Edible films and coatings in seafood preservation: A review. Food Chemistry. 2018;**240**:505-513. DOI: 10.1016/j.foodchem.2017.07.034

[23] Bekhit M, Arab-Tehrany E, Kahn CJ, Cleymand F, Fleutot S, Desobry S, et al. Bioactive films containing alginate-pectin composite microbeads with *Lactococcus lactis* subsp. *lactis*: Physicochemical characterization and antilisterial activity. International Journal of Molecular Sciences. 2018;**19**:574. DOI: 10.3390/ijms19020574

[24] Beristain-Bauza SC, Mani-López E, Palou E, López-Malo A. Antimicrobial activity and physical properties of protein films added with cell-free supernatant of *Lactobacillus rhamnosus*. Food Control. 2016;**62**:44-51. DOI: 10.1016/j.foodcont.2015.10.007

[25] Hernandez-Izquierdo VM, Krochta JM. Thermoplastic processing of proteins for film formation—A review. Journal of Food Science. 2008;**73**:R30-R39. DOI: 10.1111/j.1750-3841.2007.00636.x

[26] Wang H, Hu D, Ma Q, Wang L. Physical and antioxidant properties of flexible soy protein isolate films by incorporating chestnut (*Castanea mollissima*) bur extracts. LWT—Food Science and Technology. 2016;**71**:33-39. DOI: 10.1016/j.lwt.2016.03.025

[27] Hashemi SMB, Mousavi Khaneghah A, Ghaderi Ghahfarrokhi M, Eş I. Basil-seed gum containing Origanum vulgare subsp. viride essential oil as edible coating for fresh cut apricots. Postharvest Biology and Technology. 2017;**125**:26-34. DOI: 10.1016/j.postharvbio.2016.11.003

[28] Riaz A, Lei S, Akhtar HMS, Wan P, Chen D, Jabbar S, et al. Preparation and characterization of chitosan-based antimicrobial active food packaging film incorporated with apple peel polyphenols. International Journal of Biological Macromolecules. 2018;**114**:547-555. DOI: 10.1016/j.ijbiomac.2018.03.126

[29] Liu Y, Cai Y, Jiang X, Wu J, Le X. Molecular interactions, characterization and antimicrobial activity of curcumin–chitosan blend films. Food Hydrocolloids. 2016;**52**:564-572. DOI: 10.1016/j.foodhyd.2015.08.005

[30] Kalaycıoğlu Z, Torlak E, Akın-Evingür G, Özen İ, Erim FB. Antimicrobial and physical properties of chitosan films incorporated with turmeric extract. International Journal of Biological Macromolecules. 2017;**101**:882-888. DOI: 10.1016/j.ijbiomac.2017.03.174

[31] Han Y, Yu M, Wang L. Physical and antimicrobial properties of sodium alginate/carboxymethyl cellulose films incorporated with cinnamon essential oil. Food Packaging and Shelf Life. 2018;**15**:35-42. DOI: 10.1016/j.fpsl.2017.11.001

[32] Xu Y, Rehmani N, Alsubaie L, Kim C, Sismour E, Scales A. Tapioca starch active nanocomposite films and their antimicrobial effectiveness on ready-to-eat chicken meat. Food Packaging and Shelf Life. 2018;**16**:86-91. DOI: 10.1016/j.fpsl.2018.02.006

[33] Rattaya S, Benjakul S, Prodpran T. Properties of fish skin gelatin film incorporated with seaweed extract. Journal of Food Engineering. 2009;**95**:151-157. DOI: 10.1016/j.jfoodeng.2009.04.022

[34] Shahbazi Y. The properties of chitosan and gelatin films incorporated with ethanolic red grape seed extract and *Ziziphora clinopodioides* essential oil as biodegradable materials for active food packaging. International Journal of Biological Macromolecules. 2017;**99**:746-753. DOI: 10.1016/j.ijbiomac.2017.03.065

[35] Siripatrawan U, Vitchayakitti W. Improving functional properties of chitosan films as active food packaging by incorporating with propolis. Food Hydrocolloids. 2016;**61**:695-702. DOI: 10.1016/j.foodhyd.2016.06.001

[36] Campos CA, Gerschenson LN, Flores SK. Development of edible films and coatings with antimicrobial activity. Food and Bioprocess Technology. 2011;**4**:849-875. DOI: 10.1007/s11947-010-0434-1

[37] Kaya M, Ravikumar P, Ilk S, Mujtaba M, Akyuz L, Labidi J, et al. Production and characterization of chitosan based edible films from *Berberis crataegina's* fruit extract and seed oil. Innovative Food Science & Emerging Technologies. 2018;**45**:287-297. DOI: 10.1016/j.ifset.2017.11.013

[38] Ochoa TA, Almendárez BEG, Reyes AA, Pastrana DMR, López GFG, Belloso OM, et al. Design and characterization of corn starch edible films including beeswax and natural antimicrobials. Food and Bioprocess Technology. 2017;**10**:103-114. DOI: 10.1007/s11947-016-1800-4

[39] Andrade MA, Ribeiro-Santos R, Costa Bonito MC, Saraiva M, Sanches-Silva A. Characterization of rosemary and thyme extracts for incorporation into a whey protein based film. LWT—Food Science and Technology. 2018;**92**:497-508. DOI: 10.1016/j.lwt.2018.02.041

[40] Putsakum G, Lee DS, Suthiluk P, Rawdkuen S. The properties of gelatin film-neem extract and its effectiveness for preserving mined beef. In: Packaging Technology and Science. 2018;**31**:611-620. DOI: 10.1002/pts.2386

[41] Kaewprachu P, Osako K, Benjakul S, Suthiluk P, Rawdkuen S. Shelf life extension for Bluefin tuna slices (*Thunnus thynnus*) wrapped with myofibrillar protein film incorporated with catechin-Kradon extract. Food Control. 2017;**79**:333-343. DOI: 10.1016/j.foodcont.2017.04.014

[42] Cutter CN, Senevirathne RN, Chang VP, Cutaia RB, Fabrizio KA, Geiger AM, et al. Major microbiological hazards associated with packaged fresh and processed meat and poultry. In: Kerry JP, editor. Advances in Meat, Poultry and Seafood Packaging. Cambridge: Woodhead Publishing; 2012. pp. 3-41

[43] Beristain-Bauza SC, Mani-López E, Palou E, López-Malo A. Antimicrobial activity of whey protein films supplemented with *Lactobacillus sakei* cell-free supernatant on fresh beef. Food Microbiology. 2017;**62**:207-211. DOI: 10.1016/j.fm.2016.10.024

[44] Khezrian A, Shahbazi Y. Application of nanocompostie chitosan and carboxymethyl cellulose films containing natural preservative compounds in minced camel's meat. International Journal of Biological Macromolecules. 2018;**106**:1146-1158. DOI: 10.1016/j.ijbiomac.2017.08.117

[45] Giteru SG, Oey I, Ali MA, Johnson SK, Fang Z. Effect of kafirin-based films incorporating citral and quercetin on storage of fresh chicken fillets. Food Control. 2017;**80**:37-44. DOI: 10.1016/j.foodcont.2017.04.029

[46] Hamedi H, Kargozari M, Shotorbani PM, Mogadam NB, Fahimdanesh M. A novel bioactive edible coating based on sodium alginate and galbanum gum incorporated with essential oil of *Ziziphora persica*: The antioxidant and antimicrobial activity, and application in food model. Food Hydrocolloids. 2017;**72**:35-46. DOI: 10.1016/j.foodhyd.2017.05.014

[47] Caetano KS, Hessel CT, Tondo EC, Flôres SH, Cladera-Olivera F. Application of active cassava starch films incorporated with oregano essential oil and pumpkin residue extract on ground beef. Journal of Food Safety. 2017;**37**:e12355. DOI: 10.1111/jfs.12355

[48] Kaewprachu P, Osako K, Benjakul S, Rawdkuen S. Quality attributes of minced pork wrapped with catechin–lysozyme incorporated gelatin film. Food Packaging and Shelf Life. 2015;**3**:88-96. DOI: 10.1016/j.fpsl.2014.11.002

[49] Batpho K, Boonsupthip W, Rachtanapun C. Antimicrobial activity of collagen casing impregnated with nisin against foodborne microorganisms associated with ready-to-eat sausage. Food Control. 2017;**73**:1342-1352. DOI: 10.1016/j.foodcont.2016.10.053

[50] Kalem IK, Bhat ZF, Kumar S, Noor S, Desai A. The effects of bioactive edible film containing *Terminalia arjuna* on the stability of some quality attributes of Chevon sausages. Meat Science. 2018;**140**:38-43. DOI: 10.1016/j.meatsci.2018.02.011

[51] Zhang H, He P, Kang H, Li X. Antioxidant and antimicrobial effects of edible coating based on chitosan and bamboo vinegar in ready to cook pork chops. LWT—Food Science and Technology. 2018;**93**:470-476. DOI: 10.1016/j.lwt.2018.04.005

[52] Albertos I, Avena-Bustillos RJ, Martín-Diana AB, Du W-X, Rico D, McHugh TH. Antimicrobial olive leaf gelatin films for enhancing the quality of cold-smoked salmon. Food Packaging and Shelf Life. 2017;**13**:49-55. DOI: 10.1016/j.fpsl.2017.07.004

[53] Dib AL, Agabou A, Chahed A, Kurekci C, Moreno E, Espigares M, et al. Isolation, molecular characterization and antimicrobial resistance of

enterobacteriaceae isolated from fish and seafood. Food Control. 2018;**88**:54-60. DOI: 10.1016/j.foodcont.2018.01.005

[54] Yücel N, Balci Ş. Prevalence of *Listeria, Aeromonas*, and *Vibrio* species in fish used for human consumption in Turkey. Journal of Food Protection. 2010;**73**:380-384. DOI: 10.4315/0362-028X-73.2.380

[55] Kahraman BB, Dumen E, Issa G, Kahraman T, Ikiz S. Incidence of *Aeromonas hydrophila* and *Plesiomonas shigelloides* in Seafoods. Turkish Journal of Fisheries and Aquatic Sciences. 2017;**17**. DOI: 1309-1312. DOI: 10.4194/1303-2712-v17_6_24

[56] Alparslan Y, Baygar T. Effect of chitosan film coating combined with orange peel essential oil on the shelf life of deepwater pink shrimp. Food and Bioprocess Technology. 2017;**10**:842-853. DOI: 10.1007/s11947-017-1862-y

[57] Remya S, Mohan CO, Venkateshwarlu G, Sivaraman GK, Ravishankar CN. Combined effect of O_2 scavenger and antimicrobial film on shelf life of fresh cobia (*Rachycentron canadum*) fish steaks stored at 2°C. Food Control. 2017;**71**:71-78. DOI: 10.1016/j.foodcont.2016.05.038

[58] Carrión-Granda X, Fernández-Pan I, Rovira J, Maté JI. Effect of antimicrobial edible coatings and modified atmosphere packaging on the microbiological quality of cold stored hake (*Merluccius merluccius*) fillets. Journal of Food Quality. 2018;**2018**:12. DOI: 10.1155/2018/6194906

[59] Mohebi E, Shahbazi Y. Application of chitosan and gelatin based active packaging films for peeled shrimp preservation: A novel functional wrapping design. LWT—Food Science and Technology. 2017;**76**:108-116. DOI: 10.1016/j.lwt.2016.10.062

[60] Yuan G, Lv H, Tang W, Zhang X, Sun H. Effect of chitosan coating combined with pomegranate peel extract on the quality of Pacific white shrimp during iced storage. Food Control. 2016;**59**:818-823. DOI: 10.1016/j.foodcont.2015.07.011

[61] Arfat YA, Benjakul S, Vongkamjan K, Sumpavapol P, Yarnpakdee S. Shelf-life extension of refrigerated sea bass slices wrapped with fish protein isolate/fish skin gelatin-ZnO nanocomposite film incorporated with basil leaf essential oil. Journal of Food Science and Technology. 2015;**52**:6182-6193. DOI: 10.1007/s13197-014-1706-y

[62] Song HY, Shin YJ, Song KB. Preparation of a barley bran protein–gelatin composite film containing grapefruit seed extract and its application in salmon packaging. Journal of Food Engineering. 2012;**113**:541-547. DOI: 10.1016/j.jfoodeng.2012.07.010

[63] Lee J-H, Yang H-J, Lee K-Y, Song KB. Physical properties and application of a red pepper seed meal protein composite film containing oregano oil. Food Hydrocolloids. 2016;**55**:136-143. DOI: 10.1016/j.foodhyd.2015.11.013

[64] Vieira JM, Flores-López ML, de Rodríguez DJ, Sousa MC, Vicente AA, Martins JT. Effect of chitosan–Aloe vera coating on postharvest quality of blueberry (*Vaccinium corymbosum*) fruit. Postharvest Biology and Technology. 2016;**116**:88-97. DOI: 10.1016/j.postharvbio.2016.01.011

[65] Khalifa I, Barakat H, El-Mansy HA, Soliman SA. Improving the shelf-life stability of apple and strawberry fruits applying chitosan-incorporated olive oil processing residues coating. Food Packaging and Shelf Life. 2016;**9**:10-19. DOI: 10.1016/j.fpsl.2016.05.006

[66] Kraśniewska K, Gniewosz M, Synowiec A, Przybył JL, Bączek K, Węglarz Z. The use of pullulan coating enriched with plant extracts

from *Satureja hortensis* L. to maintain pepper and apple quality and safety. Postharvest Biology and Technology. 2014;**90**:63-72. DOI: 10.1016/j.postharvbio.2013.12.010

[67] Guerreiro AC, Gago CML, Faleiro ML, Miguel MGC, Antunes MDC. The effect of alginate-based edible coatings enriched with essential oils constituents on *Arbutus unedo* L. fresh fruit storage. Postharvest Biology and Technology. 2015;**100**:226-233. DOI: 10.1016/j.postharvbio.2014.09.002

[68] Jovanović GD, Klaus AS, Nikšić MP. Antimicrobial activity of chitosan coatings and films against *Listeria monocytogenes* on black radish. Revista Argentina de Microbiología. 2016;**48**:128-136. DOI: 10.1016/j.ram.2016.02.003

[69] González-Estrada RR, Chalier P, Ragazzo-Sánchez JA, Konuk D, Calderón-Santoyo M. Antimicrobial soy protein based coatings: Application to Persian lime (*Citrus latifolia* Tanaka) for protection and preservation. Postharvest Biology and Technology. 2017;**132**:138-144. DOI: 10.1016/j.postharvbio.2017.06.005

[70] Sogvar OB, Koushesh Saba M, Emamifar A. *Aloe vera* and ascorbic acid coatings maintain postharvest quality and reduce microbial load of strawberry fruit. Postharvest Biology and Technology. 2016;**114**:29-35. DOI: 10.1016/j.postharvbio.2015.11.019